HOT AND UNBOTHERED

HOT
AND
UNBOTHERED

HOW TO
THINK ABOUT,
TALK ABOUT, AND
HAVE THE SEX
YOU REALLY WANT

YANA TALLON-HICKS

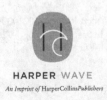

HARPER WAVE
An Imprint of HarperCollinsPublishers

FIRST EDITION

Designed by Jen Overstreet

Library of Congress Cataloging-in-Publication Data
Names: Tallon-Hicks, Yana, author.
Title: Hot and unbothered: how to think about, talk about, and have the sex you really want / Yana Tallon-Hicks.
Description: First edition. | New York, NY: Harper Wave, [2022] | Includes bibliographical references. | Summary: "A guide to investigating sexual desires, with tools to help readers communicate their wants, needs, and boundaries"— Provided by publisher.
Identifiers: LCCN 2021039630 (print) | LCCN 2021039631 (ebook) | ISBN 9780063075511 (paperback) | ISBN 9780063075528 (ebook)
Subjects: LCSH: Sexual excitement. | Sexual fantasies. | Sex.
Classification: LCC HQ31 .T267 2022 (print) | LCC HQ31 (ebook) | DDC 306.7—dc23/eng/20211013
LC record available at https://lccn.loc.gov/2021039630
LC ebook record available at https://lccn.loc.gov/2021039631

ISBN 978-0-06-307551-1

22 23 24 25 26 LSC 10 9 8 7 6 5 4 3 2 1

This book is dedicated to my clients—past, present, and future.

CONTENTS

A Couple of Brief Notes

All clients written about in this book represent composite characters and stories of clients I have worked with throughout my time as a therapist, sex educator, and advice columnist. Though the issues and dynamics portrayed in these client stories are very real, the individual people spoken about are not.

Any and all identifying details that may be true to real clients such as names, ages, locations, occupations, situational details, genders, sexualities, and relationship structures have been strategically altered in order to protect the very privileged privacy of my real clients, whose dilemmas and trust I value and respect immensely. If you are seeing yourself reflected in the client stories in this book, it is likely because the particular situations and conundrums I chose to represent are just that common, which is why I used them as examples in the first place.

All personal stories told about my own life and my past and present sexual and/or romantic partners are real but have been similarly altered to protect individual privacy and have been told from my singular perspective.

I hope that all of these stories help normalize sex and sexuality as well as the humanness, dilemmas, and solutions they illustrate.

I also want to take a few moments to make some personal acknowledgments about my identities and privileges as they relate to my work. I am white, cisgender, thin, and able-bodied. I am also a presently well-resourced queer/bisexual woman in a straight-passing relationship. I was raised in an upwardly mobile middle-class family on the East Coast of the United States and am both highly educated and gainfully self-employed. My success in my field and my access to various platforms to safely speak and write about sex are undoubtedly influenced by my racial, body, and class privilege, just to name a few. As a white sex educator and writer, I have benefited by way of white privilege[1] from both past and current[2] racist reproductive health research practices,[3] laws, and acts in this country and beyond. To not acknowledge this harm here would be to perpetuate it.

The information and perspectives I share in this book are heavily informed by my personal positions of privilege, and my perspective on these issues will be limited by these lenses. There is always more to learn about myself and my work as it and the world around me changes and evolves. As a reader, diversifying who you learn about sex and sexuality from is always encouraged. In the resource guide in the back of this book, you'll find a variety of other sex educators and writers to learn from, though I heavily recommend that you also look beyond what I have to offer.

HOT AND UNBOTHERED

INTRODUCTION

Hey! We're All Getting Screwed!
(by Sex Education)

I talk to people about sex for a living, sometimes one- or two-on-one in my therapy practice, sometimes in smaller groups of 10 to 100 in a college workshop setting, and sometimes to 500 strangers[1] in the middle of a modern art museum in Austria.

The first thing I like to do in all of these contexts is ask my audience: What did you learn in high school sex education?

The first response I always get is either dead silence or near-resentful laughter. "Nothing!" is usually shouted out first. Sometimes the period of silence is so long I start with my own example: "Well, I don't remember getting much sex education myself besides the classic condoms-on-bananas relay races. The unrealistic banana aside, I never did understand why we needed to learn how to race each other on competing teams for our future safer sex lives but hey, I wasn't making the rules." Small smatterings of laughter always break the ice and help strangers feel more comfortable talking to you about sex.

More importantly, once the people in the audience know that the *sexpert* in front of them is also a real human with her own lackluster sex education history, their own examples follow:

"That penis-in-vagina sex is the only 'real' way to have sex."
"I only learned about heterosexual people."

"STIs."

"Unwanted pregnancy."

"Abstinence only."

"We watched scary birth videos."

"I didn't have any sex ed."

"Our gym teacher was so uncomfortable we mostly talked about the weather."

Whether I'm teaching on a college campus, at a high school, or to a room full of adults in my local sex toy shop, these responses rarely change. The younger generations might utilize Google and TikTok more, sure, but the state of formal U.S. sex education seemingly hasn't evolved much. I make sure to congratulate the few younger students who boastfully tell tales of their uber-inclusive and modern Our Whole Lives (O.W.L.) programs[2] taught at their Unitarian Universalist youth groups; otherwise, in a country that only requires sex education in 28 states (15 of which are not required to present medically accurate information),[3] the responses to "What did you learn in high school sex ed class?" remain (depressingly) evergreen.

It's not like sex ed has stayed essentially the same because it's working. As of this writing, 70 percent of U.S. states have requirements to stress abstinence as the only or preferred option for safer sex,[4] and yet the United States has one of the highest teen birth rates[5] and the highest STI rate of all industrialized countries. European sex education is doing a little better, sure, but sex education in schools is mandatory in only 11 out of 25 European countries,[6] and research has reported that sex education teachers are rarely satisfactorily trained and that the classes often overemphasize biological issues, much like the sex ed taught in the States. But rarely do these classes include discussions about the relationship aspects of sex such as communication, consent, and boundaries, nor do they examine the pleasure-based aspects like pleasurable, non-reproductive anatomy such as the clitoris.

The only place that gets a sex ed cookie, in my eyes, is the Netherlands or, as my partner gracefully puts it, "Everyone's got a sex ed boner for the Dutch!" And for good reason. The Dutch begin "sex education" in kindergarten. However, you'll never hear a direct reference to sex in sex ed classes until it's deemed age-appropriate: kindergarteners start with talking about the concept of love and relationships; 8-year-olds learn about self-image and gender stereotypes; 11-year-olds discuss sexual orientation and healthy relationships. Younger students learn basic relational skills like how to ask permission, how to hear *no*, and how everyone's bodies and identities are equally valid in the wide world of relationships. They start early with this compulsory relational education, and they do so with wildly productive results. The Netherlands can brag about some of the best outcomes when it comes to teen sexual health: Dutch teens use the birth control pill more often than their U.S. counterparts[7] and they have one of the lowest teen pregnancy rates[8] in the world. On average, Dutch youth do not have sex at an earlier age[9] than those in other European countries or in the United States and, most impactfully, when they do decide to have sex, *they report the most "wanted and fun" first sexual experiences.*[10]

While most national funding programs would probably rather hear about the STI and pregnancy stats connected to sex ed, as a pleasure- and consent-focused sex educator, my "sex ed boner for the Dutch" comes from this: *the most wanted and fun.*

In the United States, we're still reeling from a booming #MeToo movement,[11] weeding our collective pop culture garden of powerful (mostly famous) sexual harassers, predatory politicians, and (sometimes serial) rapists. As this upheaval trickles down, I hear clients, students, and peers struggle to understand how this translates to our casual Tinder dates, our porn preferences, our perhaps questionably consensual past sexual experiences, and even our Netflix queues. Meanwhile, our sex educational programming continues to hinge on the message: "Be afraid . . . be very afraid."

In fact, fear continues to be the primary motivator for most sex education efforts in this country: We are taught to fear STIs and unwanted pregnancy, we inherit stigma about our masturbation habits and our sex toy collections, and we're taught to judge each other and ourselves for having too much sex, not enough sex, or the wrong kinds of sex. We're afraid to take too long to climax or climax too quickly, to buy lube, to talk to our friends and even our therapists about our kinks, to say *no* to our partners, and to say *yes* to ourselves.

Meanwhile, media depictions of sex and relationships, with their focus on all that can go poorly, have been teaching us the same fear-based attitudes toward sex. But they've been teaching us to fear the wrong things. Rather than teach us to fear a system that teaches men to equate hearing *no* with a threat to their self-worth, or a system that speaks of sex as something women "give up," men "score," and queer, trans, and LGBTQQIA+ people, apparently, just don't have,[12] we are being taught to fear what makes sex so appealing in the first place—*pleasure*.

What if, instead of being taught to fear sex, we were taught the relational skills necessary to navigate our most pleasurable—or, our most wanted and fun—sexual experiences? This is what I hope to do in my workshops, in my client sessions, in my lectures, and here in this book.

After I ask my audience what they've learned about sex in high school sex ed, I always then ask: "Where have you learned about sexual pleasure?"

"Friends."

"Word of mouth."

"Experimentation."

And then, typically a long pause.

And then, from the back of the room, a brave-yet-sheepish "Porn?"

"Yes!" I tell the audience, perhaps too enthusiastically in an attempt to quickly minimize any shame felt by the person who's called such X-rated content into the room—and because they're totally right. Research has shown that by age 18, over 90 percent of boys and over 60 percent of girls[13] have watched porn online. Twenty-three percent of U.S. youth ages 10–15 have intentionally sought out porn.[14] Fourteen percent of youth in Europe have done the same, starting as early as nine years old.[15] In contrast, the reported age of "virginity loss"[16] in U.S. teens is 17 years old[17] across the gender spectrum. This means that in both the U.S. and Europe at least, most young people are watching porn before they are having sex.

Thanks in no small part to our smartphones, porn is more accessible than ever. Now, I'm not personally anti-porn. I watch porn, I don't think all porn is bad, nor do I think it's single-handedly contributing to the violent degradation of women everywhere (but that's a different book entirely). If you look in the back of this book you'll even find a section in the resource guide devoted to my top porn recommendations. But I do think that, like all media, porn is a genre that requires viewers to have the maturity and critical thinking capabilities necessary to absorb what we are watching, register it as fantasy, make decisions about how/if the porn we're watching is congruent with our beliefs and ethics, and filter it as entertainment that is separate from our personal reality. I do not believe that a 10-year-old has the ability to do this. Especially in the context of our aforementioned sex education system, and extra especially when we imagine what types of porn a 10-year-old might find with a simple, unrefined Google search about sex.

Porn, especially in isolation, is not comprehensive sex education. But our deficit in actual, honest, pleasure-based, consent-focused, and accurate sex education[18] can make it seem like a suitable replacement. Every single young person interviewed in one Boston University study[19] reported that they were learning how to have sex by watching pornography. Specifically, what sex positions to use, how to pleasure their partner, or how to engage in particular sex acts (e.g., oral, anal, etc.)—topics that center on pleasure rather than reproduction and, as it happens, are very conspicuously left out of sex education. More informally, LGBTQQIA+ clients, workshop attendees, and personal friends have frequently told me that they turned to porn for sex education after even more progressive sex ed curricula left them unable to answer the most basic question: "How do LGBTQQIA+ people have sex?" It's not that youth are seeking out porn because it's the most appealing, approachable, or accurate source of sexual information; it is simply more readily available—and, perhaps more importantly, less hollow and less centered on scare tactics than their parents, peers, and teachers. Porn is oftentimes the only resource that doesn't send the message "sex feels bad" or "sex is bad" but sends the message (sure, sometimes dramatically) "sex feels good!" Young people are trying to learn from porn what the rest of us are failing to teach them about: sexual pleasure.

Especially if porn isn't part of your personal sexual repertoire (and extra especially if you're quite anti-porn) maybe you're wondering why the heck I'm spending so much time talking about it here in this book about sexual pleasure. Porn, and specifically mainstream porn, may be a great (or sometimes the only) place to learn about what sexual pleasure can look like, but it is typically a mediocre and often confusing place to learn about how to actually experience sexual pleasure for yourself. When we think about how sexual pleasure occurs in mainstream porn, we might encounter a handsomely tipped (wink wink) pizza delivery guy, somehow seamless shower sex (that shit is much harder in real life than it looks!), and easily and quickly synchronized orgasms (despite the fact that nearly 80 percent of people with vulvas require direct and consistent clitoral stimulation in order to climax).[20]

What we don't get to see in mainstream porn is conversation, snack breaks, boundary negotiations, STI disclosures, fumbling with condoms, hurt feelings, physical variety, giving direction to partners about how to touch you, laughing when someone accidentally smacks you in the jaw with their knee while you're going down on them, or otherwise perfectly human experiences of sex. With all of these real components missing, the essential sex educational pieces absent from porn include: consent, self-knowing, self-discovery, and how, actually, realistically, to find and experience our most authentically pleasurable sex lives.

Well, shit. So, here you are, having gotten no pleasure education from formal sex education and a warped version of pleasure education from mainstream porn. We're not bad, broken, deficient, or "bad at sex"; we've just been left in the dark about how to access pleasure, how to remove barriers to that pleasure, and how to navigate actual, consensual, pleasurable sex with our partners.

This collective frustration pops up *very frequently* in the form of questions and dilemmas from clients, sex column readers, and workshop attendees: "How do I tell my partner what I want?"; "How do I know what I want, sexually?"; "How do I practice consent without being awkward as hell?"; "Is it normal that I like X, don't want Y, or fantasize about Z?"; "I want to feel good but I don't know how to do it."; "What do we do if we don't like the same things?"; "How do I tell my partners 'yes', 'no', or 'maybe'?"; "Am I weird?"; "Am I broken?"; "Why can't I figure this out?"; "Can you help me?"

In this book, I'll do my darndest to answer all of the above questions and then some, but the short answer to the last question is: *yes*. Helping you with your sex life is exactly what I'm about to do.

Hot and Unbothered hopes to inspire you and your partner(s) to talk about, think about, and have authentically pleasurable sex without the shame, secrecy, self-doubt, and misinformation that has perhaps clouded your view of what's possible in your intimate relationships. To do this, *Hot and Unbothered* will guide you through the arc of how I design and teach my workshops about sex, sexuality, consent, and pleasure so that you can bring this sexual freedom-finding format into your own lives with ease.

In Part 1, we'll deconstruct the model of sex that's been handed to us. We'll take a good, hard look at our existing sexual resources and contexts, and the messages we've gotten from them, so that we can normalize how most of us are caught in the same, lackluster sex educational soup, one that has failed us in many ways. We'll question this traditional model that has encouraged us to see "good sex" as a box to fit into rather than as a custom container we can build to suit us as individuals. We'll also examine how this unhelpful framing of sex has convinced us that we are not worthy or capable of the sexual pleasure that is truly possible in our lives.

With the fresh perspective gained from unburdening ourselves of these stale ideas, we then begin deconstruction in earnest. In Part 2, we remove the common barriers contained in the factory model of good sex discussed in Part 1 so that we can start fresh in designing a sex life custom fit to our genuine pleasure. We will deconstruct the *Classic Mood* (Chapter 3), design our *Authentic Mood* (Chapter 3), identify our own limiting *Pleasure Pessimism* (Chapter 4), and begin reconstruction with Chapter 5, "Reshaping Negative Narratives."

In Part 3, our path to real pleasure has been cleared and the fun begins as we answer questions like: Who are we, *really*, as sexual individuals? What do we want? What do we like? What have we yet to discover? How do we want to go about exploring? Part 3 dives into these questions with "How to Discover What You Want" (Chapter 6), "How to Ask for What You Want" (Chapter 7), and "Setting Your Sexual Boundaries" (Chapter 8). Part 3 shows that whether with yourself, a casual encounter, or a long-term partner, your pleasure absolutely matters and is well within your reach.

Finally, for added pleasure security, Part 4 addresses common stumbling blocks, troubleshooting moments, and potential back-slides with "How to Hear *No* Like a Pro" (Chapter 9), "How to Repair a Boundary Mistake" (Chapter 10), and "How to Navigate Desire Discrepancies" (Chapter 11) so that you can be sure that all of your new discoveries are as sustainable as possible even after the book's last page turns.

Hot and Unbothered intends to fill the gap left behind by traditional sex educational models and casual peer-based sex education by giving you explicit permission to talk about, think about, and have authentically pleasurable sex without the shame and secrecy that has powered our deepest understandings of sex for centuries. I believe that the more casually we can talk about sex, the less shame we breed. I believe that the more we know about sex toys, kinks, orgasms, communication, our bodies, our partners' bodies, and what makes us and them squirm, the better and healthier sex and relationships we'll all have. I believe that learning how to laugh during sex will make us all more willing to take the risks that make great sex great. I believe that learning how to say an enthusiastic "Yes!" to the kinds of sex we want will make the *no*s that much easier and the *yes*es that much more valuable.

If there's anything my combined educational and personal experiences, my clients, my readers, and my peers have taught me, it's that giving ourselves explicit permission to feel good can change us, putting real effort into making others feel good is a gift well within our reach to give, and genuine pleasure can absolutely overturn our own and our culture's strained relationship with sex and consent. In the spirit of a future filled with consensual pleasure, read this book and apply its contents to your sex life only with explicit permission from yourself and only if and when it feels authentically good to you to do so. Because if it's not wanted, fun, and pleasurable, then what's the frickin' point?

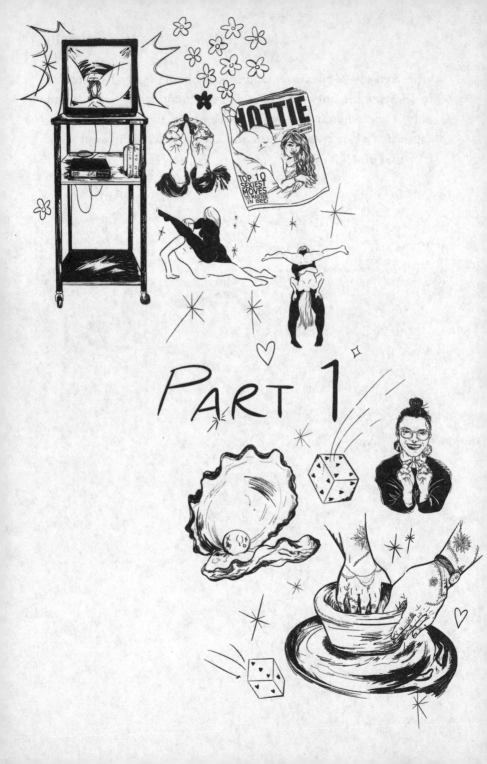

PART 1

We're going to keep it short and sweet here in Part I. In the following two chapters, you'll learn that real sex is the best sex and you'll begin to discover what the *real* in *real sex* means to you. Part I encourages you to discard the constraining, media-promoted ideas of what makes a person "good at sex," squash your own sexual imposter syndrome, and begin to clearly articulate your vision of your most authentically pleasurable sex life. Part I says good sex isn't something happening somewhere outside of your real life; rather, downright excellent sex is already set up to happen here, in your real life, now.

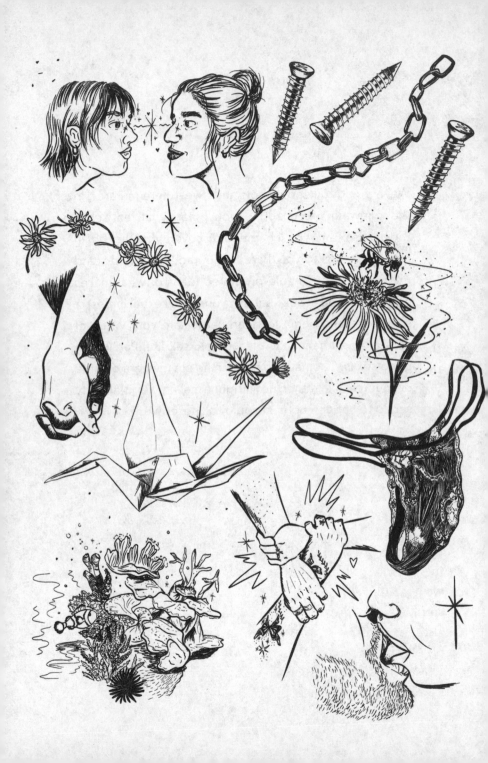

CHAPTER 1

On Good (Sexual) Relations

You are normal; it is the world around you that is broken.[1]
—*Emily Nagoski,* Come as You Are

My bed frame collapsed underneath us right around the time Lincoln started voraciously kissing my neck. "Sex so good we broke the bed frame!" someone might've reported to friends at brunch the next day. But here, on our first date, the broken bed frame was a welcome interruption, a jarring not-so-far-to-fall thud that let me pause just long enough to recognize my feeling of relief followed by my realization that, hey, I could just end this lackluster sexual experience right now.

"Sorry," I apologized on behalf of Ikea. Lincoln gallantly and very nakedly crouched down on all fours to try to figure out what exactly had cracked underneath us. "You don't need to do that," I insisted, staring at the hair on Lincoln's ass, noticing how truly naked we both were now that we were just here in my room, doing something so nonsexual as trying to fix a bed frame. "Should we just call it?" I asked, the broken mattress slats being the conspicuous cherry on top of our failed sexual sundae, which had also included one scoop of bad kissing and two scoops of completely absent chemistry.

"Sure," Lincoln responded with a look of relief so clear I knew I wasn't the only one here who was just not feeling it.

"Okay, cool. I had fun at dinner, though. I'm sorry we didn't really connect otherwise." I genuinely meant it. We had been acquaintances first with a lot of shared professional interests and some social overlap. We both really liked trying new local restaurants, and he was nice and just sarcastic enough to keep me engaged. The gnocchi, at least, had been stellar.

The problem with being a sex columnist and sex educator is that, when it comes to dating, your imagined reputation precedes you. And it's painfully obvious when it has. For example, when a first date like Lincoln randomly picks up my entire body to awkwardly hold me against the wall of my apartment to make out with me in a way that screams, "This is totally out of my wheelhouse but I saw it in a porn once!" Or when a college hook-up of mine, Charlie, made a split-second decision to pour half a bottle of water onto my head when I was giving him a blow job—*why, sir?*—in a seemingly desperate attempt to stand out from the imagined crowd of creative and brave lovers I had, in his mind, surely had before him. Another date, Kate, had gleaned from my social media that I knew a thing or two about kinky sex, and she spent so much time trying to embody a dirty-talking, bossy persona that clearly didn't turn her on or suit her, I thought maybe I had unknowingly become audience to a one-woman, erotic spoken-word piece.

Though I suppose I could be flattered at all of these sexual stops being pulled out on my behalf, it's hard to feel anything but embarrassed and disconnected when someone is having sex with you based on an image of sex they have in their minds rather than the actual sexual interaction they are having with *you*—the unique human being in front of them.

Yes, it's entirely true that I have multiple boxes of sex toys in my home, walls covered in quirky, erotic art, and a whole lot to say about things like vibrators, rope bondage, anal sex, three-somes, and non-monogamy. I am also a regular human being. I get nervous on dates, I have terrible "game," I make mistakes, I've been heartbroken more than twice, and I am not as easy to hoist up against a wall for a steamy make-out as I might appear. Most importantly, just like you, I am not sexually one-size-fits-all. I don't want to be impressed with the skills my partners think they're bringing me, I want to be *involved* in the sex we are creating together—freaky, waterlogged, bed-breaking, or otherwise.

To be clear, I did not experience my consent as violated during these awkward sexual moments.[2] And though Lincoln and I didn't date again, we kept in touch as friends. I did go on to date and have plenty of good and great sex with the other two heroes of these rough-starting stories, after we made some adjustments (more on how to make adjustments in Chapters 7 and 8). To me, these attempts at sexually performing felt like exactly that: a disconnected sexual performance, misguided by the sex education and sexual examples we get of what makes for good sex.

In the United States (and likely in some other parts of the world, I am sure), we've got a real confused relationship to our bodies, sex, and relationships—especially when it comes to the topic of feeling pleasure in any or all three. We are a country founded on puritanical morals, nonconsent, violence, capitalism, and merit-based competition.[3] And in our sex education (both formally in school and informally through family, friends, and media), these roots show.

Shame-based puritanical ideologies want to keep pleasure and the complexities of sexuality out of reach and out of the conversation[4] (think abstinence-only sex education, dropping your voice to a whisper when mentioning something sexual, using your browser's incognito mode when watching porn). Capitalism knows simultaneously that: 1) sex sells (think: every advertisement you've ever seen, from cars to hamburgers), and 2) they can't effectively sell you what you think you already have (you'll never be good enough, worthy enough, sexy enough until you have XYZ or look like *blah, blah, blah*).

From these various avenues, we inherit a big ol' contradictory mess of sex education:

- Have consensual sex but don't talk about sex.
- If you don't have X amount of sex, you're a loser.
- If you have X amount of sex, you're a slut.
- No one will have sex with you unless . . .
- Sex is always dangerous—you're either always perpetrating violence (typically messaged to men) or need to always protect yourself from it (typically messaged to women and LGBTQQIA+ folks).
- Sex is no big deal—relax and just go with it!
- No sex before marriage.
- Virgins are dorks. And college-aged virgins?? Even bigger dorks.
- Give her an orgasm (but don't ask her how).
- Make your partner feel special (but don't fake your pleasure).
- Your desire is too low.
- Your desire is too high.
- Your desire is too high about the wrong things, or types of sex, or sex acts, or partners, and it's too low about the right things, or types of sex, or sex acts, or partners.
- Fix yourself.
- You're inadequate.
- You're too much.

- 10 Sex Tips That'll Make His Toes Curl.
- Give the Best Blow Job of His Life.
- What Women Really Want!
- Are You a Sex Addict?
- Seven Secrets Hidden in the Trap Door of Your G-Spot That Will Open Up into an Even More Secret Sex Disco But Only If You Do These Three Specific Moves and Also Know the Password.

These multiple, conflicting messages come to us in a slow, eroding drip over time—in our classrooms, relationships, work commutes, magazines, social media feeds, friendships, families, movies—culminating in an internalized thesis statement that boils down to:

1. You are not supposed to want or desire sex (especially the kind of sex that really, really turns you on).
2. You need to be the best at having the most and *goodest* sex possible.
3. In other words: you must win at sex, but no, not like that.

What Makes for Good Sex

After over a decade of doing this work, I firmly believe that everybody who is interested in having sex wants to be good at it. Or, at the very least, they want to have sex that is good rather than sex that is not. Meaning, we are motivated to experience good sex and, as can be seen by the above list, we are likely often confused about how, exactly, to get there.

Dirty talking, tossing a partner against a wall in a passionate fervor, taking control, delivering orgasms, writhing around in (overblown and sometimes downright-faked) ecstasy, pretzeling yourself into a million different shapes and calling them "creative positions that'll blow her mind"—these are common pieces of seemingly pleasure-forward "good at sex" advice. But this advice won't get you far if the person you're having sex with just isn't into those things.

Advice like this sets us up to view sexual pleasure, our experience of it, and our success as sexual partners as an individual project—a solo skill set to master, applying a one-size-fits-all style to every sexual encounter. (Think: Lincoln sees hot porn dude toss hot porn lady against a wall; Lincoln decides to attempt this move on our first date.) But good sex is not that (sorry, Lincoln)— it is a living, breathing collaborative project that shifts and changes based on variables like who you're sleeping with, where, when, how you feel that day, and what you hope to get out of sex that night, as well as your partner's particular turn-ons and turn-offs, just to name a few. This means good sex is much less about *what* you're doing, and much more about *who* you're doing it with. And, because your kindergarten teacher was right and each of us is indeed special and unique, this means having good sex requires a more complex, multifaceted approach than the titillating magazine headlines might have us believe.

I don't know how to teach you to contort your body into a bunch of wild, muscle-pulling positions, but I can tell you how to have good—might I even venture, great—sex:

1. Take stock: Who are you interested in having or currently having sex with?
2. Ask them: What, for you, makes for great sex?
3. Tell them: What, for you, makes for great sex.

4. Listen to what they have to say before, during, and after sex.
5. Make adjustments.
6. Enjoy your great sex.

Though this is the truth, it's the stripped-down version of the truth. Of course, in our real lives, nothing about sex and pleasure is that simple. Shame, stigma, unhelpful self-talk about our sexuality and desires, lack of access to inclusive sex education, scarce resources, competing advice about the same topic—these are just a few of the many barriers we need to work through as we reach toward our authentic sexual pleasure. Oh, and don't forget, we're also expected to do all of this perfectly and within a very limited scope of body type, sexuality, gender, and desire. This super narrow model of being "good at sex" says, "You can't do this, as you are, with what you have, now."

I say, "Of course you can."

Good sex isn't encapsulated by how you give a blow job, your sex toy collection, your sexual resume, or what your body looks like. Good sex is actually highly subjective in the technical and material department. What I did to have mind-blowing sex with one partner may very well translate to so-so sex with the next. The only real way for anyone to know how to have good sex with anyone else is to communicate with that person about sex: to inquire about what makes sex good for them, to share what makes sex good for you, and to set the stage for said communication to happen in a safe, honest, and productive way. All of this is to say that objectively good sex is actually not defined by the technical or material; it's entirely relational.

There's a thin line between communicating well and relating well, and both are pillars of my go-to advice about how to have good sex. Don't know what your partner wants in bed? Ask. Want something new or different out of your sex life? Say so. Feel totally nerve-wracked about the process of doing that? Talk about *that* with your partner first.[5] Communication just makes for better, more fulfilling sex,[6] period. And the more comfortable we are in our sexual relationship (however brief or long-term the sexual relationship may be), the easier and more frequently the sexual communication will flow.

Good, partnered sex is first and foremost a relational act. Therefore, the act of having consensual and mutually pleasurable sex (the simplest definition of "good sex," in my mind)—whether for one, one hundred, or one thousand nights—requires us to have good *relational* (and no, not just sexual) skills.

Some relational/communication skills that might make you good at sex:

- Curiosity about your partner
- Asking questions (see Chapter 7)
- Asking permission and practicing consent (see Chapter 7)
- Soliciting and receiving feedback productively (see Chapter 8)
- Reading the room
- Active listening (see Chapter 9)
- Attention to body language and nonverbal cues
- Open-mindedness
- Resistance to snap judgments (of yourself or your partner)
- Awareness of nonverbal body language like open posture, attentive eye contact, and physical proximity
- Willingness to make and repair mistakes (see Chapter 10)
- Empathy

- Resilience (see Chapter 9)
- Consideration of others
- Effective communication (oh, we will get way into this, don't worry—see Chapters 6–11)
- Conflict resolution
- Self-awareness
- Setting healthy boundaries (see Chapters 8 and 10)
- Sharing (space, your thoughts, the vibrator)
- Bravery to show up as your full self
- Comfort in your vulnerability
- Social justice frameworks such as anti-racism, anti-sexism, and anti-transphobia, just to name a few
- Making requests or direct asks (see Chapter 7)
- Adaptability

Some technical skills that can *help* you be good at sex (but cannot make you good at sex *on their own*, in isolation):

- Knowledge of sexual anatomy, sex toys, erogenous zones, positions, and sexual activities (see the resource guide!)
- Knowing how and where to research sex educational questions you might have
- The resources to get and maintain sexual health screenings, treatments, and preventable measures

Some things that *do not* determine how good you are at sex (especially in the absence of any of the above):

- What your body looks like or how it functions
- The size, shape, or functionality of your genitalia

- Medications and supplements sold to you that promise instant results
- The lingerie you have on
- The music you have playing
- The number of candles you have lit
- Your sex drive
- Your age
- Your sexuality
- Your gender
- What you do for work (i.e., if you work as a sex educator, sex worker, or sex therapist)
- The number of partners you've had
- The number of times you've had sex or been sexual
- The amount of porn you have consumed
- What kind of position pretzel you can bend into
- Whether or not your ex thought you were good at sex
- The number of orgasms you or a partner have had
- How long you last
- How hard you can go
- How much your sex life mimics media-made sex lives or what your friends tell you they're up to between the sheets

The good news about relational skills is that we all know how to do at least some of them well and we can all learn how to improve the rest (if only just a little). Which means that we are all—yes, ALL—capable of having good, if not totally mind-blowing, sex. Here. In our real lives. No bedside bottles of water required.

Your Brief Guide to Consent
(and Why It Makes You Better at Sex)

If some of this chapter's relational skills for good sex are sounding a lot like the components of sexual consent practices, well, you'd be right. Though we'll dive much deeper into consent practices in Chapters 9 and 10, this couldn't be the start of a guide about authentic sexual pleasure without at least a mini 101 on active sexual consent, especially because sexual consent 100 percent includes good relational skills, and vice versa. Consent is absolutely a multifaceted, developable skill that doesn't just make for ethical and legal sex,[7] but also for good, great, excellent, and even amazing sex. Here's how:

1. Check in with yourself. What do you want? What do you not want? What do you desire? Knowing your sexual self before sexually engaging with others can make you a clearer communicator, a more confident lover, and a genuine sexual partner.

2. Check in with your partner. What do they want? What do they not want? What do they desire? Nobody said you have to come in with all of the answers about what makes your partner sexually tick and, in fact, assuming that you have them all might very well make for quite bad sex. It's always better (and, honestly, more efficient) to have a roadmap to someone's pleasure.

3. Ask your partner for their explicit permission before any and all sexual interaction (physical, verbal, over text, etc.) and wait for a verbal response. Not only is this the basis of sexual consent, but creating an opportunity for your partner to state their boundaries creates safety, trust, self-empowerment, and relaxation—all key physiological components[8] to sexual pleasure for most people.

4. Cross-check verbal responses with physical cues. Attuning to someone's body language during sex is a skill that can be practiced over time in and outside of sexual scenarios. If someone is saying, "Yes, I'm into this" while they are simultaneously looking away, physically shrinking themselves, shutting down, or otherwise physically saying, "No" or "I'm unsure," that's a great time to stop, check in, reflect on what you're seeing, and make sure green means go. It's very important to note that **this does not work in the reverse**. If someone is verbally telling you *no* and you believe you are seeing or "getting the vibe" of *yes*, that's predatory, pre-assaulting behavior. Don't do that.

5. Make sure consent is ongoingly obtainable and that all sexual activities remain optional. Many of us have heard the educational phrase "consent can be revoked at any time," and know that if given once, it doesn't apply to all sexual interactions thereafter. In order to make this so, drugs and alcohol should be avoided if and when they may make it impossible for any involved party to ongoingly obtain consent or opt out of the sexual interaction. With or without substances involved, if you can't understand someone's yes/no/maybe or freely say yes/no/maybe, ongoing consent is no longer

possible. Being able to make adjustments, change your mind, feel your pleasure, and update your consent status moment to moment is a foundational piece of good sex.

6. Talk consent to me. Check in about what's going on during sex, as you're doing it. This doesn't have to be like "Please sign here before we do X" for every single act. Rather, telling someone what you want, asking them what they want, and getting live feedback can be organic, genuine, and super hot.

7. Accept feedback and correct course. The consent process doesn't end when the sex does. Ask your partner how it went. Tell them how it went for you. Talk about the sex you had as you're sweaty and spooning right after sex and also talk about the sex you had days or weeks ago (if the relationship type allows) to make sure everything is settling okay with less adrenaline and more space. If something went awry, know that there are several available ways to correct course including changing behaviors, editing sex acts, making small adjustments, or, in some cases, engaging in an accountability or restorative justice process.[9,10] (We'll talk more about making mistakes and repair in Chapter 10.)

The Good Sex Dilemma

With all of these messages pushing us in one way and pulling us in another, it's easy to get caught up in the tug-of-war of what I like to call the Good Sex Dilemma—the place where we feel caught between what we actually want out of sex (what would truly make it uniquely good for us) and what we've been told makes for good sex. The Good Sex Dilemma is a confusing, contradictory place where many of us stand and wonder, how do I get where I want to go from here? One of my clients who found himself caught in this place is Evan.

Evan is a hipsterish type in his mid-twenties. He's got a progressive liberal arts education and has a social organizing career in his near future. Evan is my "typical client." Meaning, he came into my office with an intermediate understanding of consent-forward sex, cares earnestly about the genuine pleasure of his sexual partners, and has spent a considerable amount of pre-therapy time unpacking toxic masculinity and what it means for him to operate as a cisgender, straight man in any given social or sexual interaction.

And yet, he has not been spared the lurking confusion that can come from the onslaught of mixed messages delivered to him by formal and informal sex education about what might make him good at sex. Though he originally started therapy with me to "process some past sexual interactions," the Good Sex Dilemma has emerged as the distillation of his sexual discomfort.

For various reasons—emerging from general life circumstance, healing from heartbreak, questioning his own sexual value—sex has taken a backseat in Evan's life for the last two years. During this sex break, Evan decided to attend therapy to explore some of these issues and what might be blocking him from sex, which, he's recently admitted, he's starting to actively avoid.

Now, six months in, after we've talked weekly about his relationship to porn, his sex education from school and family and friends when he was younger, and a full history of his past sexual relationships, a new potential partner, Taylor, has just entered the picture and Evan is about to put his in-session insights to real life work.

> **Evan, at the top of our 6:30 pm session:** Well, I'm pretty sure I'm going to have sex tonight. I'm going over to her house right after this.
>
> **Me:** Alright. How do you think it's going to go?
>
> **Evan:** I'm feeling pretty good about it, feeling pretty good about it . . .
>
> **Me:** Seems like a long way to come for someone who just told me they feel "a pit of darkness open in the bottom of their stomach when faced with sex."
>
> **Evan, laughing at his own dramatic phrasing being quoted back to him:** I just want to be good at it—the sex, that is.
>
> **Me:** Sure, I think that's a very reasonable thing to want.
>
> **Evan:** But I just get so caught up in worrying about the other person, like, the person I'm having sex with. I worry about how they're feeling and what they're thinking and what they're feeling and if things are feeling good for them. On top of that, I worry about myself and how I look and how I feel and if things are feeling good to me. I feel like all of that distracts me from the sex part and then I'm not good at it.
>
> **Me:** Okay, let me just make sure I'm following you correctly. So you think that being aware of and invested in your own and your sexual partner's experience of the sex you're having together makes you . . . *bad* . . . at sex?
>
> **Evan, having a little chuckle at the reframe:** Okay, you got me.

Though I wish sex therapy could be wrapped in the neatly tied bow of a snappy reframe, it rarely ever is. But it is a good start. It can be a lot of work to untangle and reprogram deeply infiltrated messaging about sex and sexuality and what makes us "good" at it. In our previous sessions, Evan has been a really active client and has often talked openly and honestly and reflectively about sex, sexuality, masculinity, racism, and heteronormativity. And still, here we are, catching automatic thoughts and associations that have linked good sex to a specific set of knowledge and skills so often that they are still here, dictating Evan's lived, sexual life and sexual self-confidence.

We continue Evan's session with conversation about what beliefs he holds about what might make him good at sex:

- Knowing everything about sex when he walks in the door
- Being able to perform this knowledge flawlessly on anyone's body at any time
- Being unwaveringly confident in his abilities and body
- Emulating what he's seen in mainstream porn, where bulky, directive white men are generally the ideal (an ideal not reflected by Evan's body)

Then, we compare these beliefs to what kind of sex he actually wants to have:

- open
- honest
- pleasurable
- consent-forward
- gender-affirming
- feminist
- adaptable to the moment
- authentic to who he is

It becomes clear very quickly that the good-sex parameters that have been handed to him do not fit the lived experience of sex he'd like to create. Instead, his ideal lived experience of sex will be best created with communication, consent, and self- and other-awareness—*during* his date with Taylor.

Good sex cannot be created *before* Evan interacts with Taylor but rather will be co-created *as he interacts with her.* Of course, doing a live improv show can feel much scarier than a scripted show you've rehearsed a million times. This is why, as certainty-loving humans, we gravitate toward articles like "50 Tricks to Break His Sex Brain"—they make us feel rehearsed, prepared, and ironed out, like we know what the hell we are doing. But we don't. If we want to have truly good sex we've got to first acknowledge that we really don't know how to have sex with a person until we're navigating sex with that person. The best we can do is be open and excited to take the risk of finding out. This is where good relational skills come in. Good relational skills are sexually relevant skills that you can hone by yourself, then pull from your tool kit as needed while you build your custom-made sexual interactions with your partner, in real time. For Evan, the relational skills we highlighted for him to carry to that night's sex date included:

- ✔ Comfort in his own vulnerability of feeling rusty at sex and self-conscious about his body
- ✔ Asking Taylor questions about her boundaries, desires, and limits, with the help of a Yes/No/Maybe List (see Chapter 6) that he shared with her over text before they met up
- ✔ The willingness to make mistakes and see this first sexual encounter as a getting-to-know-you starting place for their (hopefully) future and ever-improving sex dates

✔ Transparency about his hopes for their sex date, which
   included a lot of communication before, during, and after
   sex, as well as a time to learn about each other and feel
   sexual pleasure while they're at it

Of course, Evan is not the only client I have battling the Good
Sex Dilemma. Annie is in her mid-thirties and suffering from vagi-
nismus, and thinks she can't possibly have good sex until she
"fixes herself." Joy and Julia are a married couple in their 50s
who have fallen into a sexual rut after years of unsuccessfully
attempting to recreate the sex life of their 20s, patterns that just
don't fit who they are as a couple and what they want out of sex
today. Kira (who we'll see in Chapter 8) has spent years thinking she needs to enjoy and have reliable orgasms from standard,
vanilla sex with her husband when all the while, it turns out,
kinky sex is really what turns her crank. Lyla's boyfriend wants
to explore receiving anal sex but Lyla is frozen in fear because
she doesn't single-handedly know every little thing about anal
sex and thinks she needs to before she and her boyfriend explore together. And Suzie believes that in order to have good
sex with the men she dates, she needs to have a showy, theatri-
cal climax every time, whether or not she's actually feeling that
much pleasure.

All of these clients share the Good Sex Dilemma in common
with the unifying threads of their internalized, unspoken beliefs
about good sex: *I need to be perfect before I can have good sex. I
need to know everything before I can have good sex. I need to have
had good sex before I can have good sex again. I need to figure this
out by myself or, at least, not with my sex partner.*

Conveniently, these problems also share the same solution:
talk about your shared sex life, with the person or people you are

sharing it with. It is well-researched that communication about sex (coupled with the perceived safety in the relationship) is a primary predictor for a subjectively satisfying sex life.[11] Specifically, open communication[12] about each partner's likes, dislikes, preferences, and desires translates directly to having a sex life that includes the things that you like and excludes the things you don't. Because we are all constantly evolving sexual creatures, good sexual communication also includes making sure that we are continually updating ourselves and the people we have sex with on the evolution of our likes, dislikes, preferences, and desires. Basically, if you want to have good sex, you have to know how to talk about good sex (i.e., have an understanding of terms and pleasurable anatomy, the comfort to discuss these things, a way to describe your desires, etc.) and actually talk about what good sex means to you.

Very well-known vulnerability and shame researcher Brené Brown clearly links shame and silence together[13] as co-conspirators in repressing our emotions, self-expression, and connection to others. It is not a far jump from there to look at the ways sexual shame and lack of communication[14] hinder us from having the sex life of our dreams. Your unhelpful personal beliefs about sex, fueled and reinforced by confusing sex ed messages, are preserved by your automatic thoughts[15] about sex, sexuality, and yourself as a sexual person as well as by your silence about sex and desire (more about transforming unhelpful automatic thoughts in Chapter 5). Something that's amazing about being a sex therapist is witnessing firsthand the near-instant transformation that can happen for clients just by speaking their sexual fears, automatic thoughts, and limiting beliefs about sex out loud. And if you can then manage to speak these things out loud to your partner(s)? That's good-sex magic.

Partnered sex is not a solo project. You bring things to it, of course! But you are not the only person in the room. You are together, with someone (or someones, as the case may be), in a sexual space and all parties involved are thinking, feeling, trying, failing, braving, enjoying, and processing all kinds of things alongside you.

This means you don't have to be flawlessly prepared, you don't have to know everything, you don't have to pull out all of the stops, and the highly subjective success of your sexual interaction doesn't all rest on your shoulders or . . . other body parts. Instead, you can ask questions, introduce something you've historically liked, teach your partner(s) about your body, Google something you don't understand yet, make a mistake and grow from it—the possibilities are endless when we defocus on being "good at sex" as a title to achieve and refocus on good sex as a relational connection, no matter how many strings are or are not attached.

Don't misunderstand me; saying "Good sex is relational" does not require you to be in a relationship or to be emotionally entangled. All you have to do is care about having sex that is good, consensual, and pleasurable to all parties involved (as you should!) and the rest will follow. The orgasms and the positions and the handcuffs and the lingerie will come (if you want it to). This can happen in a casual sex moment by asking your new sex mate:

- How do you want me to touch you?
- Does that feel good?
- What do you want next?

Moving toward relationally good sex can happen in your casual or serious relationship by asking questions over coffee or text or dinner like:

- How's our sex life been for you lately?
- I've been thinking a lot about [insert fantasy or new thing you'd like to try]. What do you think?
- I've really been loving XYZ about our sexual connection these days.

This can happen by reading your sexual partner(s)' body language and asking:

- You seem [to love when I . . . / uncomfortable when I . . . / disengaged when . . . / really into it when . . .]. Do you want [more/less/something different]?
- Do you want to take a break?
- How are you feeling?

And all of this can be positively reinforced by responding to your partner(s)' answers

- with curiosity rather than judgment.
- knowing that your partner is sharing something about themselves rather than a criticism about you.
- without self-defense or sex-shaming.
- with observable actions that reflect their requests for adjustments (with your consent, of course).[16]

Though Lincoln and I just didn't have the chemistry to justify working on our very brief sex life, Charlie and I, as well as Kate and I, absolutely utilized the above questions, communication skills, empathy, body language, checking in, open-mindedness, and curiosity to hone our shared sex craft. By utilizing good relational skills, we were able to move past the water bottles and the faux-kinkiness to develop, improve, and collaborate on our sexual interactions moving forward. It took some guess-and-test, it took some (literal) feeling out, and it didn't always look like a flawless X-rated scene, but it did make for sexual connections that were genuine rather than performative, authentic rather than canned, and co-written by us rather than dictated by a magazine's Top Tips.

When I saw Evan at our next session, he was glowing. He told me all about how much the Yes/No/Maybe List had helped him and Taylor break the ice over communicating about sexual desires and boundaries and how the entire dynamic between them seamlessly shifted from a solo good-at-sex mission to shared, authentic sexual cooperation. And because of this, for Evan as an individual, and for Taylor and Evan as new sexual partners, there was all of this available space for a fresh cycle of sexual relating to unfurl, an exciting prospect to say the least.

At the end of that night's session, Evan ended his therapy hour in the way I wish all of them might. "Wow," he said, looking down at his hands and then up at my face with a smile, "it feels so freeing to not feel the pressure to be perfect at this."

For Goodness Sex

A worksheet about which relational and communication skills make for authentically good sex, to you.

1. Do you have a favorite memory of good or even excellent sex, full of mutual pleasure? List below some elements of that really great sexual experience. No memory of good

sex to pull from? Use this list to create a wish list. I've made some category suggestions to help you along.

This is how I felt about my partner:

This is how I felt about myself:

This is how my body was feeling:

This was the vibe between us:

I could describe the sex as:

I communicated to my partner about the sex we were having/ about to have/had by:

What helped me communicate in that moment was:

What helped me feel safe in that moment was:

This is where and when we had sex:

This is how we had sex (positions, sex toys, other logistics):

This is how I had been feeling that day, in general (zoom out a little—what else was going on for you in your life generally and/or that day)?

Other:

2. What do *you*—unique human being with your own values, body, needs, boundaries, desires, and sexual history—thinks makes for good sex?

3. What components of your good sex experience from Question #1 can you easily recreate?

4. What technical skills or components of great sex do you want to learn more about or practice?

5. List some ideas about how you'd like to learn more about or practice these components (this book's resource guide can help).

6. What sexual-relational skills do you want to continue to practice?

7.   What relational skills do you want to learn more about or add into your sexual repertoire? (Hint: return to my list of some relational skills that might make you good at sex on page 10.)

8. Now, lastly, please finish the following two sentences for me:

It's important to me to be a good sexual partner because . . .

I deserve authentically pleasurable sex because . . .

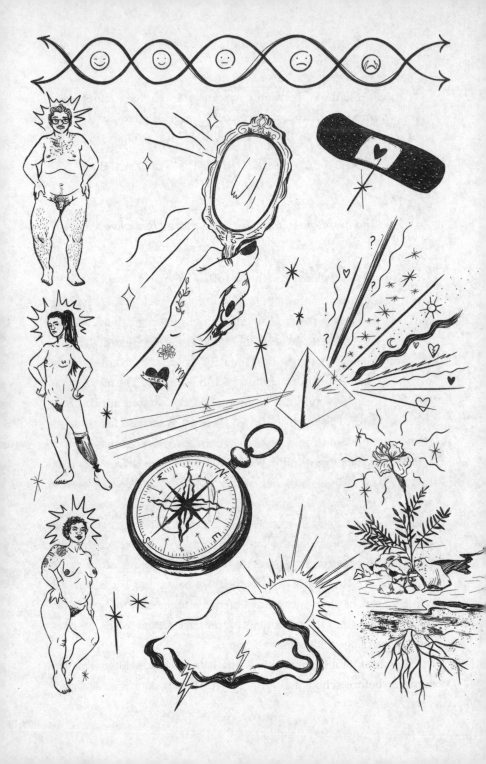

CHAPTER 2

Your Perfectly Imperfect Sex Life

The more I feel imperfect, the more I feel alive.[1]
—*Jhumpa Lahiri,* In Other Words

I was a sex columnist and sex educator long before I was a therapist. I spent my early and mid-twenties waiting tables, writing pun-heavy advice for others' sexual conundrums, and bringing bulging (sometimes vibrating) tote bags of sex toys to college campuses to teach workshops about sex and pleasure. The more popular my workshops became, the more people started approaching me afterward to ask me if I offered therapy. It seemed funny to me that anyone would consider me such an esteemed advice-giver to want me as a therapist but it also made sense, of course—you can't toss a dildo into an audience at a sex workshop without hitting at least *somebody* with some sex-related baggage to unpack. As these post-workshop inquires grew, my satisfaction in my current working life shrank: my feet were increasingly sore after my late-night serving shifts, I was starting to envision the kind of stable life structure that could accommodate a baby, and I was quickly running out of shits to give about the temperature of a wealthy stranger's coq au vin. I enrolled in graduate school to get my master's in marriage and family therapy.

My first official graduate school class was held online the summer before school actually started. It was an ethics and professionalism course that covered professional standards of the therapy field including codes of conduct, privacy and confidentiality rules, and a little exercise about public image and personal disclosure that amounted to "Go Google yourself and see what comes up. Now, write a reflection paper on what a potential client might think of what they find." I already knew full well what would be found if and when a future therapeutic client Googled me: hundreds of sex columns peppered with F-bombs and silly dildo jokes; published personal stories about topics such as my failed non-monogamous relationships or my finicky vagina's response to homemade lube I made in my kitchen once; pictures of my smiling face holding crates of sex toys with my tattooed arms and buzz-cut hair; a TED Talk that kicked off with me telling a story about watching a $5-bin porno on DVD—all things I had yet to see on a "shining example of a professional therapist" poster.

Yep, the imposter syndrome kicked in real quick.

Imposter syndrome can be summed up by the feeling and belief that "Everyone else is better and more deserving than I am. Oh, also, I'm definitely a fraud." It is often context-specific (I'm an imposter at this job, in this role, at this conference, in this friend group, in this grad program) and can come on very suddenly. Imposter syndrome is almost always felt by people who are, actually, quite qualified, who *do* have the experience and knowledge to contribute to their fields, and who were absolutely accepted into their programs, positions, or accolades by legitimate channels. In fact, imposter syndrome, by definition, is a *misplaced* fear that you are in the wrong place, for the wrong reasons. Regardless of their actual expertise and worth-validating facts about themselves, those suffering from imposter syndrome still think "I'm not as good as the people around me," "I'm not qualified, I'm faking it," "My success is a product of random luck and nothing more," and "At any moment surely someone will find me out for the imposter I am." Seventy percent of people[2] say that they have felt imposter syndrome at least once in their lifetimes. As (now famously) told by Neil Gaiman, even Neil Armstrong[3] (first man on the moon, maybe you've heard of him?) battled with imposter syndrome.

Traditional imposter syndrome is well-studied, TED Talked about, and written about in the professional realms of business, education, and research. It has a list of symptoms including anxiety, lack of self-confidence, comparison to others, negative self-talk, fear of failure, fear of future success, dwelling on the past, and lack of confidence in one's instincts and intuition. Sound sexually familiar? If this level of self-doubt shows up for 70 percent of us in our work, studies, and relationships to our professional peers, it makes perfect sense that it would also show up in our sex lives. I often hear long confessional stories from clients expressing crushing doubts, rampant self-comparisons, and a yet-to-be-recognized belief that "Sure, everyone else is allowed to explore their desires and pursue their best sex life but the same is not true for me." They're feeling what I'd like to label *sexual imposter syndrome*.

Sexual Imposter Syndrome

Sexual imposter syndrome is a specific feeling of fraudulence that shows up as a deeply rooted disbelief in our ability to have the sex we actually want to have. Like traditional imposter syndrome, sexual imposter syndrome is built on fear, self-comparison, systemic oppressions,[4] and imagined perfection. Like the Good Sex Dilemma, it's heightened by the lack of diversity in bodies, identities, and sexual scripts portrayed in mainstream porn and media.[5] If the Good Sex Dilemma has us feeling torn between the sex life of our dreams and the contradictory, traditional model of good sex, sexual imposter syndrome keeps us stuck there as it whispers the lie that you have to be perfect at the thing or different than who you are before you can do the thing.

This mode of thinking is often automatic and unchecked, and hinders people's sexual explorations of themselves. People suffering from sexual imposter syndrome avoid any chance of perceived sexual failure like the plague and either don't give themselves the opportunities to prove their fears wrong at all or, if they do, take all mistakes and imperfect humanness as evidence of their sexual fraudulence. This can lead to mistakes feeling much more devastating than they are, unrealistic expectations that leave us disappointed, and low sexual self-esteem and confidence. Sexual imposter syndrome can also have negative relational effects such as keeping couples stuck in a sexual rut longer than they'd like or preventing many from speaking up, learning, and growing in their sexual experiences. Basically, sexual imposter syndrome can keep us from having the sex we really want.

In my work, I see sexual imposter syndrome show up in a lot of ways for a lot of different clients. Nick is in his early thirties and can no longer get or maintain an erection due to a vehicle accident. Though in his email to me he tells me that he knows full well that there's an entire world of sex out there that doesn't revolve around penis-in-vagina penetration, he's still holding himself back from dating for fear that he'll be perceived as inadequate and, in his own words, as "damaged goods."

Evan, from Chapter 1, fears that he won't be fulfilling his successful sexual role as a cisgender man if he takes things slow and asks a lot of questions. He feels pressure to perform flawlessly and to know everything about his new sexual partner before he even walks in the door.

Sophie is a married mother of two, living in a small liberal arts town. Though she and her husband have agreed to shift into an open marriage so that she can explore her emerging bisexual desires, she tells me, "I hear about other women in my community who are my age who are exploring sex and intimacy with women for the first time but I could never pull that off." When I ask her why they can but she can't, and who made that rule, she can't come up with a concrete answer.

Mark and Lisa haven't had sex for four years. When I ask each of them what their biggest fear would be if they were to leave this session with plans to immediately go home and have sex today, Mark says, "That I wouldn't be good." Lisa says, "That I might want to stop in the middle if I'm not feeling it." Neither says, "I don't want to have sex with him/her" and both agree that they want to rekindle their sex life.

Emmett has consistent orgasms when they masturbate alone but experienced their first orgasm during *partnered* sex 13 years ago and has never again since. Though they describe to me over a decade's worth of colorful sexual experiences that they've earnestly enjoyed, they always punctuate them with a faked orgasm because, they told me, "It feels much more comfortable for me to perform the orgasms than to let my partners experience the disappointment of a failed sexual encounter."

These are just a handful of stories I've heard from clients. If you're seeing yourself in any of them, it's because they carry the most common structural narrative I hear: "Who I am, as I am, is not good enough, is not perfect, is not capable, and does not belong in my picture of sex. I am a sexual imposter and my human flaws and inevitable failures will expose me for the disposable fake I am. I'm scared. So I hide, avoid, turn off, and stay passively complacent about whatever form my sex life has presently taken."

Many readers may find that they have fallen into the sneaky little trap of sexual imposter syndrome. You'll know you're there if, when you think about your vision of authentically good sex, you find yourself trading one black-or-white standard (good or bad sex as outwardly determined) for another black-or-white standard (good or bad at the sex I actually want to have). If you do this (and many of us will), then you are still internalizing a specific perfect sexual standard to measure yourself against. This sexually perfect standard might not look the same for all of us—some of us might see sexual perfection as mutual, simultaneous orgasm, others as being able to get our partners off every time, others as having sex four times a week, others as having a reliable and long-lasting erection, and others as being easy-breezy about sexual adventures like group sex, non-monogamy, or kink.

Whatever your particular sexually perfect standard looks like in your imagination, take a moment to write about it in the worksheet below so that you can see what you're working with in terms of the bar you've set for yourself. Labeling and naming our hoped-for standards both lets us know what we're reaching for and can help us more accurately identify sexual imposter syndrome if it creeps in as a result of not quite achieving it.

My Perfect Sexual Standard

A quick check-in with yourself before we continue. The perfect sexual standard I'm currently dreaming of:

Looks like:

Feels like:

Includes sex acts like:

And includes the following goals:

And in this version of sexual perfection:

I am (what are you doing/saying/feeling/wearing/putting out there?):

My partner(s) is/are (what are they doing/saying/feeling/wearing/putting out there?):

If we get too attached to our imagined gold standard vision of sexual perfection, sexual imposter syndrome can be quick to stop us in our tracks to authentic sexual pleasure as we measure our real selves against our flawless fantasies. Luckily, by applying the traditional concept of imposter syndrome to our sex lives, we can pull from the suggestions that imposter syndrome researchers and psychologists recommend[6] to stop it from taking over:

1. Speak it out loud.
2. Reframe your failures.
3. Bolster your strengths.
4. Seek out representation.

5. Ask for help.

6. Reimagine success.

We'll tackle some of the more advanced approaches more thoroughly in Chapter 5, but first we must start with reimagining sexual success altogether. Instead of viewing sex as successful because it has fit neatly into our imagined parameters of sexual perfection, let's create a new bar: sex that is good and successful sex *because* it prioritizes what is real (and sure, sometimes flawed) over what is packaged, predictable, or performative. This kind of sex isn't perfect but is perfectly imperfect; it's sex that starts with us in all our humanness. Envisioning our sex lives as fluid, evolving landscapes of learning and discovery, rather than as a well-honed performance of an imagined ideal, allows us to easily and immediately cast ourselves in our vision of good sex—not "once this" or "after that" but *now*— unwashed hair, mismatched underwear, and novice nervousness be damned.

When we reimagine good sex as sex that is perfect because it starts with and includes us, as we are, we give ourselves permission to start exploring genuine pleasure with less internal resistance blocking our way. On the other hand, if we continue waiting for our sexual selves to be "enough" or otherwise void of imperfection and learning moments, we risk remaining stuck in sexual imposter syndrome for a lot longer as we disqualify ourselves from our best sex lives before we've even started. To resist falling prey to sexual imposter syndrome and the "perfect" horse it rode in on, we have to take down two of the most common and foundational pillars of this sexual self-sabotage: the myth of sexual perfection and the fear of sexual failure.

Reimagine: Authentic Sex, Not Perfect Sex

Authentic sex is fundamentally pleasurable sex. It's not pleasurable because you learned some sexual choreography from the pages of a magazine that you're now performing, complete with a standing ovation every time. Authentic sex is pleasurable because everyone involved has the safety, the language, the consent practices, and the understanding of their own desires and anatomy to communicate what feels good to them and what doesn't. Authentic sex is customized to suit the individuals having the sex they're having, and it happens in real time. This means that it's rarely predictable, pretty, or pristine. Your authentic sex life will not be perfect, and that's okay.

Having authentic sex means having preferences, limits, and opinions about sex. Many of my clients get stuck thinking that they are high maintenance, too picky, a burden, or weird for having special requests or circumstances that they bring into sex. The reality is that *everybody* is a custom-job sex partner whose best sexual experiences will be the ones that are tailored to fit them. *Everyone*. Everyone has their list of "things you should know about me before we have sex," has past experiences that influence their current sex lives, makes mistakes, has questions, changes their mind, doesn't know everything, or might not be able or want to do everything. Often, when we do go to have sex, many of us skip over these conversations or pretend that they don't need to exist (lest we come off as inexperienced, unsure, "broken," or "weird"). As a result, we end up having less-than-pleasurable sex, accepting what we get instead of asking for what we want, and faking orgasms, connection, and satisfaction as a result.

Authentically good sex is good because it is real and makes adjustments in consideration of reality. This means that real sex and even amazing sex includes:

- Trial and error (I want to learn about your and my own pleasure in a hands-on, real-time way.)
- Awkward moments (We aren't sure what we're doing yet, but let's try and modify as we go.)
- Unsure insecurities (I'm willing to go outside of my cushy comfort bubble and test my fears to take an exciting and nerve-wracking sexual adventure with you.)
- Stop-and-start pacing (We are not machines, we are real people. We might need to pee, drink water, answer a call from the babysitter; or we might get triggered or just plain tapped out.)

All of this means that an imperfect sex life actually *is* perfect because it includes *you*, a perfectly imperfect human being, and it also includes *your* genuine pleasure, not a mimicry of somebody else's. It also includes *collaboration with your partner* instead of competition with an idealized (and often fictionalized) image of what someone who is good at sex is supposed to be. Reimagining successful sex as authentic, and therefore inherently imperfect, can liberate us from sexual imposter syndrome, a crucial step toward building our most pleasurable sex lives. The standard notion of good sex places around our sex lives a limiting box that has been pre-constructed for us by external factors. When we start exploring our authentic desires, bodies, and sexual experiences, we might look at ourselves and then look at this good-sex box and think, "Dang, this is a real square peg–round hole situation—I'll never fit into this." By shedding sexual imposter syndrome, you can pull apart this pre-fab good-sex box, keep what serves you, toss what doesn't, and use the new materials and tools in this book to build good-sex parameters that are custom-made to suit *your* body, *your* desires, *your* partners, and *your* relationships.

By customizing our sexual containers, we give ourselves the freedom to modify our concept of successful sex as many times as we'd like. This means that our idea of sexual success can change as we change because our bodies, boundaries, wants, relationships, and sex lives will inevitably shift over time. And when they do, rather than saying, "I don't fit into this anymore" (sexual imposter syndrome at work) we say, "This version of my/our sex life no longer serves me, let's make some alterations" (embracing authenticity).

This reframing of successful sex is almost always my first step as a sexuality professional, and I see it work with my clients daily. Like with Nick, Evan, Sophie, Emmett, and Mark and Lisa, this reframing of sex frees people of the glue keeping them stuck in their unsatisfying sex lives, allowing them the crucial space to explore, play, imagine new possibilities, experiment, and create a rejuvenated (and attainable!) sex life they truly desire.

For example, Mark and Lisa, like many long-term couples, came to me in the state of a sex drought—a four-year sex drought to be precise. The last time they had a regular, consistent sex life, Mark and Lisa had been trying for two years to conceive their youngest daughter. Though their conception-focused sex life was self-described by both Mark and Lisa as "enjoyable," they agreed that this now-historical drive for sex was powered by their mutual desire to have another child. Though they were over the moon to add a healthy and thriving baby to their family four years ago, that was when the sex stopped entirely.

Like most long-term couples, Mark and Lisa wax poetic about a former sex life ripe with orgasms, spontaneity, mutual desire, exploration, and synchronicity. Both of them wonder openly about "what happened" and take guesses that center the blame on themselves: "I'm just so tired and shut down," says Lisa. "I don't want to do anything she doesn't want to do so I just don't bring it up at all anymore," says Mark. Lisa says, "I want to want to have sex, but I just don't," and Mark says, "I'd be excited to have sex if Lisa wanted to but I'm also scared it wouldn't go well."

Well, what does *go well* mean, anyway? Mark and Lisa have a shared concept of what their good sex-life standard looks like based on their former, pre-children sex life—a sex life that also took place in the context of their relationship being new and exciting to both of them, padded by far more free time and less stress. Their sex life used to be spontaneous, mutually desired, easy, and hot. They would both be in the mood for sex at the same time, the passion was smoldering, and the timing was always right. Some things about Mark, Lisa, and their relationship have changed since then: two babies, pelvic floor injuries for Lisa during their second baby's childbirth, fear of a third accidental pregnancy, increased work stress and pressure for Mark, a tiring household full of demands from two young kids, a ripening relationship that's full of a little less mystery and a lot more history. Like everyone's will, Mark and Lisa's sex life circumstances have changed. But what has yet to catch up with these changes is their concept of what makes for good sex.

Without updating their shared vision of good sex, it's easy for both Mark and Lisa to feel like sexual imposters. Because they both have the idea that what makes for good sex is sex that is fiery, spontaneous, physically easy, and casually coordinated like they had at the start of their relationship, it's all too easy for each of them to assess their capacity, bodies, and energy levels now and think, "I can't do that," "I'm not going to reach those expectations," "I'm going to disappoint my partner," and "I'm no longer good at sex." Instead, Mark and Lisa need to take stock of where they are today, what each of their desires are now, and how they are going to ease back into custom-building an updated version of their sex life using all of this current information.

To start the conversation about sexual imposter syndrome with couples who consider themselves stuck in a sex rut (and there are so many), I like to ask, "What would be your biggest fear if you were to leave this session today with plans to immediately go home and have sex?" As I mentioned previously, Mark answers, "That I wouldn't be good," and Lisa responds, "That I might want to stop in the middle if I'm not feeling it and we'll both just end up disappointed." Neither says, "I don't want to have sex with him/her" and both agree, "We want to rekindle our sex life but aren't sure how." What these answers tell me is that Lisa and Mark are looking to run a marathon today without having even gone for a light jog at any point in the last four years.

And this is exactly what I tell them: "You're expecting entirely too much of yourselves if feeling rusty at sex isn't allowed in your sex life after a four-year break. Of course you don't want to have sex if that's the bar. It's way too high and isn't going to set either of you up to feel successful. Instead of going from zero to sixty, why don't we try going from zero to five? What does five look like?"

In answering this question, Mark and Lisa are able to think about who they are and what they want out of sex, *today*. Their new good-sex goals include setting aside intentional time for intimate connection, heavy amounts of foreplay, a blanket expectation that they can and likely will stop and start, space for mistakes and re-learning about each other, and leaving out penis-in-vagina intercourse entirely for now. It also includes the understanding that these initial, post–dry-spell sexual interactions will change, evolve, and act as building blocks for their future, more easygoing sex life with time and practice. With this new vision of sexual success, both Mark and Lisa feel their sexual imposter syndrome lift. They have adjusted their standards away from their former sex life and toward a sex life that actually suits them. This lowered pressure increases Lisa's desire for sexual connection with Mark, increases Mark's belief in his own sexual abilities, and sets a new precedent for continued customization and newness in their shared sex life moving forward.

Of course, none of this goes perfectly. And in fact, doing this kind of work with sexual partners requires us to expect mistakes, learning moments, and failure. Because of this, one of the important pieces of our work together is to shift Mark and Lisa's relationship to anticipate failure so that failure becomes a productive and maybe even welcome friend instead of a feared foe.

Reimagine: Failure Is Your Friend

We can't talk about good sex without talking about bad sex. Or, more specifically, the fear of what might make us, personally, bad at sex. Fear of sexual failure recurs in almost all of my clients' stories—it's at the root of their sexual imposter syndrome and is offered as an explanation of why they are avoiding sex, not speaking up during sex, not initiating sex, and generally not even having conversations with their partners about sex at all.

As I've mentioned before, it's my observation that people who value sex tend to also value being good at sex. When these values are paired together, we create specific standards for what we believe makes us good at sex or what qualifies as a good sexual experience. When we worry that we might not meet those standards (remember, most of us, at some point, will not), we can automatically feel fear and shame and their close behavioral companions, silence (not speaking up about what we want or asking our partners what they want) and/or physically shutting down (freezing, avoidance, fleeing, or numbing out).[7] We tend to do this subconsciously and accidentally as we do our darndest to cram ourselves into our predetermined good-sex parameters even if our actual experiences don't fit within them.

Fear of failure isn't exactly an aphrodisiac for most. To paraphrase Emily Nagoski in her excellent book *Come as You Are*[8] about the science of pleasure, fear is a feeling that activates our lizard brain, the physiological response rooted in our survival-based, animalistic origins that screams, "WE GOTTA GET THE FUCK OUT OF HERE; THERE'S A LION IN THOSE BUSHES." In response (here, the lion is sexual failure), some of us freeze and play dead, some of us become hypervigilant in preparation to flee, some of us numb out and hope the lion kills us quickly, and some of us opt for a combo pack.

None of these responses have our bodies and our minds saying, "You know what I really want to do now that I know this lion is hunting me? Lay back and enjoy some relaxing cunnilingus." What a fear of failure *does* is shut down our bodies, create a lack of sexual confidence, discourage us from communication, and impede us from taking healthy sexual risks. Basically, fear of failure is not going to help you communicate nor climax, my friends, so let's try on a different relationship to it.

If we are to invite amazing sex into our lives, failure needs to be welcome to join the party. Especially if we are to shift focus away from a goal-oriented vision of sex to an authentic, pleasure-oriented vision of sex, we need to make friends with failure—both real failure (we tried this new sex thing and it did *not* pan out) and imagined failure (omg omg omg what if I tell my partner about this fantasy I have and he thinks I'm a total freak?). If we don't fold the possibility of failure into our idea of what makes for good sex, we remain stuck in a fear-based place that not only activates that lizard brain, but can act as a real libido-crusher. For most people, unless they eroticize fear (and there are plenty of safe, consensual ways kinky folks do this—see the resource guide), it acts as a desire and sex repellent.

Happily, the research on combating traditional imposter syndrome[9] offers us some effective ways to think differently about failure that are easily applicable to our sex lives and the fear of failure that can come with sexual imposter syndrome:

1. View good sex as a spectrum of dynamic experiences rather than as a binary pass/fail performance.
2. Move away from a fixed mindset and toward a growth mindset.
3. Learn and practice new strategies to build resiliency to failure so that when it does happen, you can bounce back quickly and refocus on pleasure.

Failure Reframe #1: Successful Sex Is on a Spectrum

If I was out on a date with someone with the agreed-upon and mutual intention of having sex together and, before knowing anything at all about me or my body, this person declared "Baby, I'm going to rock your WORLD in the sack TONIGHT!" I would be highly skeptical (and likely very turned off). First, despite what they think they're communicating, people who blow this kind of hot air about their sexual prowess aren't exactly saying, "I care about your genuine pleasure" or "Baby, I'm going to ask the most THOUGHTFUL QUESTIONS about your sexual interests TO-NIGHT!" Second, this kind of blanket-statement bravado about one's presumed future sexual accomplishments is hard to believe, seeing as so far they've completely left you (the other very important half of this sexual equation) out entirely. Unless they were boasting about their excellent sexual communication skills and real-time flexibility to shifting desires and boundaries, I wouldn't buy stock in it.

Truly successful and mutually pleasurable sex cannot be deemed so by one partner and certainly not before any communication about sex has occurred. Customized concepts of sexual success start with you and your partner(s) and are built from the ground up, not with a gold-standard ideal that was handed to you from the top down. Authentic, built-from-the-ground-up sex has a much greater chance of being more pleasurable sex because it is tailored to you and your partner(s) rather than being tethered to a perfect ideal you think you must satisfy.

The toxic idea of "perfect" sex is typically based on a goal-oriented view of sex, created *before* considering the current needs and desires of the partners involved. This kind of sex can easily become wrapped up in one partner's ego quest to prove sexual prowess and tilt into just plain bad sex. It demands, "Validate me!" instead of asking, "What feels good between us?" and yells, "Look at this!" instead of asking, "What do we want to create today?" Can you be confident in and maybe even brag about your sexual skills? Absolutely! But let that confidence be based primarily on the alternative, less-considered sexual skills listed in Chapter 1 such as empathy, active listening, willingness to be corrected, resiliency to setbacks, and an ease with your sexual body and desires, not with how hard, fast, or long "you can go."

Sex is not an Olympic sport judged on objective technique and success. There are no judges hiding in your closet waiting to hold up a scorecard. Authentically pleasurable sex is an imperfect process of discovery—of yourself and your partner(s). This means, happily, that imperfect sex is not bad sex. And actually, bad sex is usually just an ego project with a communication problem—easily avoided if you're paying attention.

Reflection: Successful Sex Is on a Spectrum

Of course, good sex isn't *one hundred* percent relational. Good sex involves a multitude of skills, from knowing sexual anatomy and positions to practicing technical aspects of sex acts, as well as relational skills like communication, attunement, knowing yourself, and feeling deeper confidence in yourself, your body, and your boundaries. A performance-based idea of good sex can often overstate the importance of skills and events ("I give such good head!", "I'm the best at cunnilingus!", "You'll orgasm twenty times with me!") and undermine the importance of customization, asking questions, and listening to what your partner wants ("What's your favorite part about getting head?", "Are you into cunnilingus?", "Are orgasms important to you and if so, what's your favorite way to have one?").

To right this balance between technical and relational sexual skills, let's do an exercise where we refocus on how successful sex *feels* rather than what it achieves.

I Know That Sex Was Successful If I Feel
(Circle all that apply and please do add your own.)

Before

Safe	Interested	Curious	Turned On
Excited	Intrigued	Well Matched	Happy
Joyful	Silly	Empowered	Desired
Liked			

Your additions here:

During

Hot	Turned On	Safe	Comfortable
Curious	Excited	Exciting	Pleasured
Pleasuring	Confident	Desired	Playful
Sexy	Adventurous	Taken Care of	Spiritual
Powerful	Submissive	Dominant	In the Moment

Your additions here:

After

Sleepy	Independent	Satisfied	Comfortable
Relieved	De-stressed	Curious for More	Intrigued
Thirsty for Knowledge about a New Sex Thing	Like I Learned Something New about Myself	Like I Learned Something New about My Partner	Heard
Seen	Understood	Connected	Loved
Joyful	Emotional		

Your additions here:

Failure Reframe #2: Adopt a Growth Mindset

A fixed mindset of sexual success views any given sexual interaction as an isolated pass/fail, good/bad event. Conversely, approaching sex with a growth mindset looks at every sexual interaction (even the smaller interactions within one sexual interaction) as a fluid experience that builds on the previous interaction, adds to your library of sexual knowledge about yourself and your partner(s), and teaches you something new about who you are as a sexual person.

Though this can be most easily conceptualized in the context of an established, ongoing sexual partnership (We learned something new about our sex life the last time we had sex, so now we can make edits and adjustments the next time we have sex), this can absolutely apply to casual sexual relationships and even one-night stands. Consider going into every sexual experience you have with the questions "*How* can I rock your sexual world, baby?" and "How else can we have fun in the event that our sexual worlds are not rocked but enjoyably rolled instead?" Though almost every chapter in this book will offer you realistic questions to ask and directives to give, some great ones to start with are "What do you want?", "I would love to . . . ," "How do you like to be touched?", "I like this, not this," "May I . . . ?", "Will you . . . ?"

Starting sex with this kind of curiosity and flexibility opens us up to countless possibilities beyond pass/fail and good/bad. When we allow ourselves to stay stuck in a fixed mindset[10] place, we set ourselves up with a limited outcome—either this sex was good or it was bad, either I'm good at sex or I'm bad at sex, this experience was either a success or a failure. This mindset only worsens our sexual imposter syndrome, layers on the sexual shame, and can even impede our desire for sex entirely. Instead, a growth mindset acknowledges that real sex isn't always simply defined by binaries like amazing or meh, achieved or in-progress, or even satisfying or unsatisfying, but can actually be both messy *and* good, both smokin' hot *and* a learning experience, both nerve-wracking *and* confidence-boosting.

A growth mindset gifts us this "both/and" reality of sex, which then gives us permission to make mistakes, to learn a new skill, to try, and to fail, without making permanent judgments about ourselves, our abilities, or our sexual worth. This creates more space for experimentation, for healthy sexual risks, for sexual pleasure, and for authenticity while also keeping us connected to our sexual partners and their real pleasure as well. Rather than containing your sexual story within the bookends of one sexual interaction, a growth mindset of sexual success looks at each sexual interaction as a piece of the unfinished story, to be continued with much more fun, learning, and excitement.

Reflection: Adopt a Growth Mindset

Chances are, you've already been shifting into a growth mindset about your sex life on your own. I mean, why did you even pick up this book? What are some of your sexual goals, hopes, and curiosities? How are you hoping this book will propel you toward this new big picture of sex?

Three things I want to learn about my sexual self are:

1.

2.

3.

Three things I want to learn about my partner are:

1.

2.

3.

Something I thought I had permanently failed at in my sex life is:

Emmett's example: Being able to climax during partnered sex.

1.

2.

3.

4.

Two ways I could revisit and explore that "failure" is:

Emmett's example:

1. Tell my next partner honestly if I've climaxed or not, without judgment of myself or of them.

2. Practice verbally stating what I want to my next partner to see if that makes partnered climax more possible for me.

1.

2.

Failure Reframe #3: Build Resilience to Failure

If we tell ourselves something enough times, we start to believe it. This has a ripple effect on the way we feel about ourselves and the world around us and how we behave in our relationships, both intimate and platonic. This is the simplified basis of cognitive behavioral therapy (CBT)[11] and its goal: cognitive restructuring. Change the way you think, says CBT, to change the way you feel and act. Though we will dive further into how to use the strategies offered by CBT to improve your sex life in Chapters 5 and 11, I want to mention some basic cognitive restructuring tricks that can be useful tools in building your resiliency to failure in your sex life, both real and imagined, now.

Fear of sexual failure can take all shapes—fear of disappointing our lovers, fear of asking for too much, fear of being "too finicky," and so on—and these fears can be based in reality (this thing I fear happened in real life once or several times and now I fear a repeat performance) or it can be imagined (what if this, what if that). Fear of sexual failure can keep many of us stuck in a sexual rut and block us from communicating with our partners about the sex we actually want to have, which can then also bar us from experiencing our most pleasurable sex lives. Fear of failure can also make us act closed off, performative, or otherwise disingenuous in our partnered sexual interactions, which decreases connection, impedes the feeling of safety and openness in our sex lives, and creates barriers to sexually collaborating with our partners. And finally, fear of failure lays a solid groundwork for sexual imposter syndrome to keep us stuck.

CBT is one of the most empirically researched forms of therapy, backed by many evidence-based studies[12] that show its impact and effectiveness. It's used to treat common client concerns like anxiety, depression, and other mental health struggles through identifying a client's automatic, unhelpful thoughts and restructuring them to create more hopeful and positive outlooks. Much of the research on resilient people[13] (those who bounce back from setbacks and disappointments easier than others) shows that they have certain cognitive structures (or schemas) that are entirely teachable to and adoptable by others who do not have these resilient cognitive structures already.

This is great news because it means that you, too, can shift how you view and relate to failure in your sex life, clearing the way to a more fulfilling sexual experience. Truly shifting our cognitive structuring around sexual failure will take time, practice, and, for some, extended work with a therapist, but there are some helpful strategies that you can hit the ground (or the bed) with now such as thought awareness, response choice, and perspective taking that can absolutely be applied to how you think about failure in your sex life, today.

From what we know about the cognitive structures and thought processes of generally resilient people, sexually resilient people may do one or many of things in their sex lives, especially as related to real or imagined failure. The following list describes a few of the perspectives commonly used by people who have resilient mindsets.

Resilient Mindsets

- See failure as a challenge, not as a reflection of your sexual worth. Just because *something* didn't work doesn't mean *you* don't work. Try a new thing that flopped? Get creative about ways to troubleshoot. Read a book about the thing, take a class, or dust yourself off and try, try again. Don't forget to have fun.

- View failure as impermanent rather than permanent. Resilient people maintain a positive image of the future and believe in their capacity to learn and change. Rather than talking to yourself in absolutes, shrink the severity of your perceived failure and put it in perspective. For example, instead of thinking, "I suck at being the dominant one, I'll never be able do it!", tell yourself something like, "Trying out a new dominant persona in bed didn't work for me this time, but that doesn't mean I can *never* take on the role of the dominant partner in bed. Here are some things I'd like to learn about or do differently next time."

- View sexual interactions as they come (or as they don't come, as the case may be). Resilient people don't take one experience and apply it as a general rule to all similar experiences henceforth. Never say never (and never say always, for that matter). Instead, find joy and freedom in customizing your sex life to every new sexual partner and even to every new day with the same sexual partner. Let your failures reflect on the growth edges of the sexual moment, not on the entirety of your sex life or sexual selfhood.

- Only attempt to control yourself and how you respond to failure rather than try to control the failure itself. People who lack resilience can be self-flagellating perfectionists, quick to assign permanent and judgmental blame to themselves or their partners. Or, less resilient people can take the opposite approach—they view themselves as simply helpless to their failed circumstances. Resilient people consider multiple, contributing factors to sexual failure, accepting what they can't change and creatively solving what they can for a more empowered approach.

- Treat your partner(s) with empathy and compassion while maintaining your own sexual selfhood. Fear of sexual failure can lead some people to bend their boundaries in order to please others or avoid disappointment. A resilient approach maintains confidence in your boundaries and resists shame if you and your partner(s)' desires simply don't line up (lots more on this in Chapter 11). When you keep your boundaries intact and true to yourself, your sense of self also remains intact regardless of how "well" the sexual interaction went. This way, you can resist equating, "That wasn't the best sex ever" with "I'm just bad at sex and will be forever."

- Maintain an ongoing commitment to your most pleasurable and authentic sex life. As Emily Nagoski says, "pleasure is the measure."[14] Repave your way toward sexual success as a leisurely, winding path through pleasure and experience, not as a superhighway that you competitively race down to your performance-based goals.

- Approach your sex life with intention and respect. Resilient people have a solid vision of what they want in various areas of their lives and have a genuine desire to put in work and effort toward achieving their dreams. When failure pops up, view it in the context of the big picture of your sex life and how this learning moment fits into the overall sex life you want to create.

Reflection: Build Resilience to Failure

Practice makes perfectly imperfect. Here we'll try on a new way of thinking that's proven to build resiliency to failure using an example from your present-day sex life.

1. Everyone's got at least one experience of real (this thing happened) or imagined (what if this thing happens?) sexual failure. List one of yours here:

Sophie's example: What if I go out with a woman in my town and people gossip and/or don't take my marriage to my husband seriously, making my sexuality exploration a foolish joke?

What's yours?

2. Now, choose one of the bullet points from the list of resilient mindsets (in the preceding text) that resonates with you and write it down here:

Sophie's resilient mindset: Only attempt to control yourself and how you respond to failure rather than try to control the failure itself.

Your resilient mindset (see bullet-pointed list on pages 57–59):

3. Apply this resilient mindset to your feared failure and write down some possible alternative ways of thinking about the fear you listed in response to #1.

Sophie's example: I can't control what people will say or think in response to seeing me out on a date with a woman, especially in a small town like mine. What I can control is being sure in my desire to explore my sexuality, confident in my marriage and my husband's consent to our arrangement, and remember that enjoying my date is the goal, not managing the rumor mill of everyone around us.

Your resilient reframe:

Reimagining Your Sex Life

Sexual perfectionism and fear of sexual failure keep many trapped in the perspective that sex is a fixed, independently curated experience that's either good or bad, successful or not, possible and permissible, or impossible and taboo. I have seen this binary and fear-fueled, defeatist way of thinking about oneself, sexuality, and the act of sex itself limit many clients and advice seekers for far longer than necessary. Don't take a back seat in your own sex life, letting your fears prove you right. Grant yourself the bravery and flexibility to try on a new perspective, a new position, or that new piece of leather you've been eyeing. Venture out and gather new evidence contrary to your fears of failure and imperfection as you go. Sex is a shared, custom-built experience with joys, flaws, and fails that takes place between perfectly imperfect humans, each with their own unique skills, baggage, and growth edges.

Nervousness, self-doubt, and even embarrassment are temporary emotional states that can absolutely mingle with pleasure, excitement, and satisfaction and, for most people, are part of the complete package of authentically good sex. Nobody knows everything about sex, is inherently good at everything about sex, or feels like they've always done everything exactly the way they hoped they would during sex. Meaning, once again, you are normal and you belong here in your imperfectly perfect and ever-evolving sex life.

When we adopt this reality-embracing, both/and perspective in our sex lives, we redefine sex as perfectly imperfect, failure as a friend, and we internalize some new truths about our sexual selves: I can have amazing sex and not be perfect. Mishaps and unknowns are part of the universal sexual experience. I deserve pleasure over perfection. I'm good enough to create my best sex life right now.

Getting Unstuck from a Sex Rut
7 Steps to Rehydrating Your Sex Life after a Dry Spell

You may be stuck in a sex rut if you and your partner(s) want to have more frequent and/or different types of sex than you're currently having but you can't seem to figure out how to do so. For some people, even the idea of sex has fallen by the wayside. Here is a small step-by-step guide to getting unstuck, which can be expanded and deepened with the guidance of a sex therapist.

1. Label that rut! Talk to your partner about the sex rut. More often than not, if you feel like you're in a sex rut, they do, too. Partners who find the most traction in getting out of their sex rut can openly agree on feeling stuck and can say to each other, "We are stuck! And we want something different!"

2. Set your goals. What does your unstuck vision of sex look like? Consider frequency, duration of sex, content of sex, types of sex, and each of your desires, limits, and boundaries. Don't assume that either or both of you want to have the same sex you were having before you hit your rut. Chances are, you don't.

3. Discuss barriers to your ideal vision of sex. What do you think is keeping you stuck in a sex rut? Is there a pattern you notice

that needs to be broken? Collaborate on some creative ideas to change that pattern, even if just a little. (Also read more about scaling barriers to sex in the upcoming chapters.)

4.   Make a starter list. Brainstorm a list of easy ways you can try new things together, break unhelpful patterns, or re-introduce sex into your lives. Make this starter list easy to achieve and keep your expectations realistic. Remember, like Mark and Lisa, you'll be more inclined to avoid sex if you're trying to go from zero to sixty and more confident in getting sexually started again if you're aiming to go from zero to five. What is your five?

5.   Set a date. Either schedule a time for sex on your calendar or schedule a window for more spontaneous sex (for example, at some point this week, one of us will initiate sex). Though scheduling sex has not been shown to us as the sexy ideal, for most partners and especially for partners in a rut, waiting for sex to spontaneously occur can result in a longer-than-desired wait time for sex!

6.   Make a backup plan. A lot of partners feel nervous or hesi-tant to restart sex because they fear it won't go "perfectly." You're probably right, so plan for that. If something doesn't go according to your plans or hopes, have some backup ideas handy that will keep you connected to each other during the time you set aside for sex: if trying something new, revert to tried-and-true sex favorites; transition to massage; take a bath together; or just cuddle and watch a movie. Adopt flexibility and stay connected whether sex happens or not.

7. Redefine success. Getting unstuck from a sex rut rarely happens overnight and generally doesn't happen after one attempt at rekindling sex. Most partners will have to strike their match more than once to get a fire started. Instead, look at this new prioritization and collaboration around rekindling your sex life as progress in itself, because that's exactly what it is.

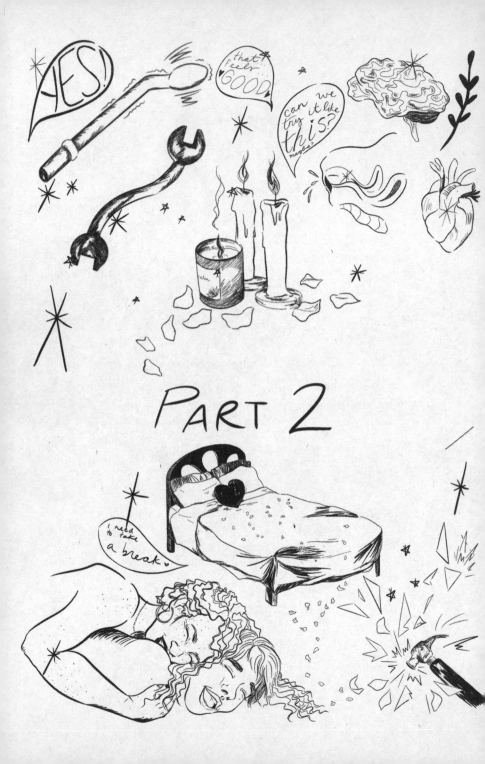

Part 2 presents and dismantles the most common barriers that I see standing between most of my clients and their genuinely pleasurable sex lives. the Classic Mood, Pleasure Pessimism, and Negative Narratives. This section of the book is all about unraveling the harmful ways we've been conditioned to think about our sexual selves in terms of where we belong, what we deserve, and the mutually satisfying sex lives we can create. These chapters include therapeutic interventions and plenty of worksheets to help free you from these pleasure-limiting, thought–action patterns. I suggest you grab a pen.

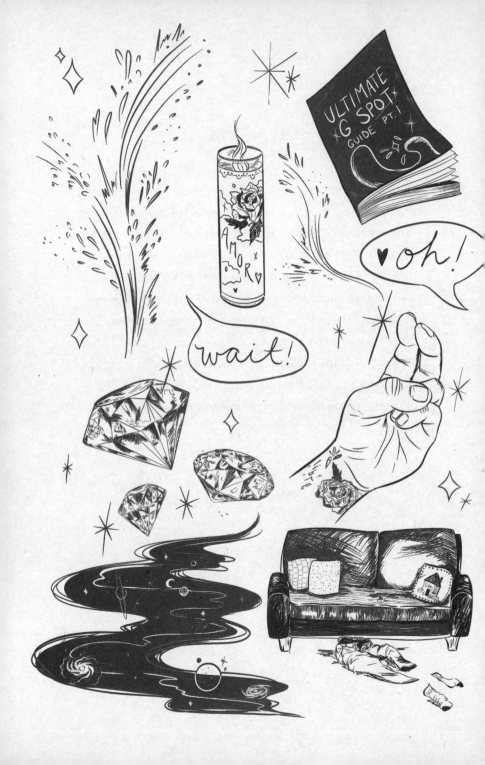

CHAPTER 3

Barrier #1: The Mood

Sexuality is one of the ways that we become enlight-ened, actually, because it leads us to self-knowledge.[1]
—*Alice Walker*

I was a teenager when I accidentally found my G-spot. Well, tech-nically, my boyfriend found it, but let's at least call it a collabo-rative effort. It was the early 2000s and the time was *teenager sex o'clock*—that precious, debaucherous 90 minutes between when you get home from school and your parents get home from work—and we were enjoying a roll in the hay (meaning, his parents' couch). As an older teen, my sexual career had really just gotten started so I didn't know much, but I knew three things for sure:

1. I truly desired the sex I was having.
2. I felt undeniably safe with my boyfriend.
3. Whatever he was doing at that particular moment felt re-ally flippin' good.

I gave what little direction/feedback I could muster ("What-ever you're doing . . . feels . . . great . . .") and then the proof was truly in the puddle, as I unexpectedly and joyously vaginally ejaculated all over the living room couch cushion. "Whoa, what?? What was that? It felt . . . awesome!" I managed to choke out between breathless breaths. "I don't know!" he said. "But my mom's going to be home in like 10 minutes."

Teenagers rarely have time and space to bask in the afterglow, so we were no slouches when it came to jumping up and furiously pulling our jeans over our sweaty legs whilst troubleshooting my curious sexual mess. "Flip the cushion over!" "It soaked through to the other side, dude!" "Okay, I think my sister has a hair dryer." "Does she happen to have two? Where are your outlets?" Bless the thick-haired sisters of this world because nine minutes and two hairdryers later we were sitting on a (mostly) dry couch cushion, staring in the general direction of a TV show when his mom walked in the door.

As teenagers, we rarely have the resources to be *too* particular about setting "the mood" (what with *teenager sex o'clock* and your parents' couch and all) but, like most elements of the brand-new world of young sexuality, we do develop certain ideas of what "the mood" might be and that we must, at all costs, avoid "ruining" it very early on.

Whether we're pulling from PG examples set for us in movies or if we've braved the world wide web of mainstream porn, most of us are left with a generally similar understanding of what I like to call the *Classic Mood*. Depending on the variation of the Classic Mood you're going for, there may be a variety of components: candles, lingerie, maybe sex toys, or if you're on a mainstream porn set: shower sex with your sky-high stilettos still on, of course.

Though the setting of the Classic Mood might change, the way we're "supposed to" communicate and act within the Classic Mood stays the same: we're intuitively connected to our partner's body and desires, we make no mistakes, and we certainly don't offer any constructive feedback or correction—we exist solely in our perfect, physical, sexual bodies, and we definitely don't pause, talk, or, Sex Lords forbid, fart. The Classic Mood is here to dictate our sexiness, and our actual needs or impulses could "ruin it" at any moment.

When I tour high schools and colleges, I ask students why they don't practice active, verbal consent more often in their sex lives, especially if and when all of them agree that it's an important thing to do. "It will ruin the mood" or "It's awkward" (another mood-ruining state-of-being) are always the first answers given. When adult clients of all ages come into my therapy office and tell me that they're not having the kind of sex they want to have, or that they're not experiencing pleasure during sex, or that their partner is doing something between the sheets that just isn't doing it for them, I ask them, "How do you give your partner this feedback during sex?" Most of them stare at me like I have a dildo stuck to my face, like why would my sex therapist suggest such a mood-ruining thing? We'll get into the specifics of how to give feedback a little later, but first let's break down the Classic Mood.

At its most basic, the Classic Mood convinces us not to talk about sex before, after, and certainly not during sex. The Classic Mood tells us that if we just light enough candles, we will have set the stage for sex so perfectly that the rest will naturally, word-lessly follow. The Classic Mood expects us to build our sex lives around the question "How can I experience sexual pleasure without saying one word about what actually brings me pleasure?"

In our efforts to not ruin the Classic Mood, what we are actually ruining is our chance of having our most genuinely pleasurable sex life.

Wellllll fuck. Now what?

This is exactly where my teenage boyfriend and I found ourselves days after my accidental couch cushion G-spot gush—now what? As newly sexual teenagers, we really just didn't have the resources to communicate about or recreate our excellent accident (also mind you this was in the early days of the Internet, before smartphones and social media, so we definitely didn't have access to the information that could've helped us). When it comes to the Classic Mood, all happy sexual accidents are exactly that—an accident. Without information, or feedback, or talking about our sex lives as they're happening, it's harder for us to record what worked for us and why, let alone figure out how to repeat it. Without permission (internal or external) to try and possibly fail, we fall prey to the Classic Mood and maintain barriers between ourselves, our partners, and our authentic sexual pleasure.

I was in my early twenties when I found my G-spot a second time, which, incidentally, was also when I found it for good. This time I had a few more clutch elements at my disposal: I was a little older and a little wiser about my own body and sexuality. And, as an extreme bonus, I had an overflowing wealth of accurate and empowering information about sexual pleasure available to me. It was 2009-ish and I was living in San Francisco and working at iconic feminist sex toy store Good Vibrations as a sex educator/ sales associate, a job where I not only received 16 hours of professional training about sex, sexuality, sex toys, and pleasurable anatomy, but also had unlimited access to an entire, carefully curated library of books and DVDs about sex. Armed with the light and easy-to-read instructional book *The Good Vibrations Guide: The G-Spot*[2] and the determination to recreate my teenaged couch cushion experience, my girlfriend and I set up shop in our tiny studio apartment.

"I know that I can vaginally ejaculate. I did it once by accident when I was younger. But I can't figure out how to get myself to do it," I told her. At this point in my sex toy–selling career, my girlfriend was used to me bringing home entire cardboard boxes of unwanted sex toy samples, slightly defective dildos unfit to sell, and employee-discounted vibrators, books, and lubes to try at home. I opened the book to a specific page that featured an internal anatomical map of the G-spot. "See?" I said, pointing vaguely as I stripped off my clothes. "That's where it is." Bless the good-natured, can-do girlfriends of this world because she barely batted an eye at my suggestion that we treat rediscovering my G-spot orgasm like building a step-by-step Ikea dresser.

Your Mini-Guide to Pleasuring the G-Spot

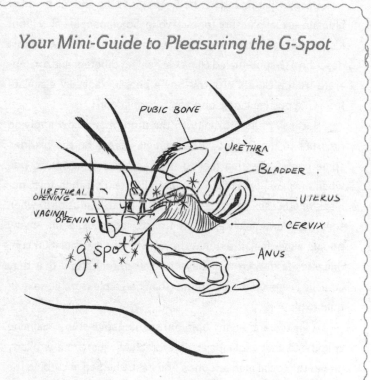

The G-spot is said to be named after German physician Ernst Gräfenberg[3] who wrote about the existence of this pleasurable little patch in the 1950s. The G-spot is located about two knuckles deep (that's not very deep!) on the inside front wall of the vaginal canal and is most easily reached and stimulated with a curved object or a position that angles your chosen penetrative object toward that zone.

The area of the G-spot can be described as rigid, spongy, or differently textured than the rest of the vaginal tissues surrounding it. (I like to compare it to the way the roof of your mouth might feel if you briefly burned it with the hot, bubbling cheese of a piece of pizza you got too excited about eating.)

Despite its reputation, the G-spot isn't the end-all, be-all of ultimate sexual pleasure for everyone. Some people enjoy it but it's not their favorite, some find the sensation irritating, and most describe a G-spot–fueled climax as feeling different and/or separate from a clitoral orgasm. Some people vaginally ejaculate from G-spot stimulation, and some people don't.

Because of its proximity to the urethra and how applying pressure to the G-spot can sometimes press on the bladder, some people describe feeling the sensation of having to pee when their G-spot is being stimulated either by hands, toys, penises, or other sex-safe objects. This has led to confusion if/when some people vaginally ejaculate from G-spot stimulation—many people either feel afraid that they might pee if stimulation continues or (if they've vaginally ejaculated) feel afraid that they actually just peed the bed rather than had a pleasurable sexual-fluid explosion.

A limited and (in my opinion) sex-negative study[4] claiming confidently that vaginal ejaculate is actually just urine regularly makes the social media rounds and hasn't helped in curbing the belief that it's just pee, leading vaginal ejaculators everywhere to either fear, disbelieve, or invalidate their own sexual pleasure. Several sex educators have banded together via the Twitter hashtag #notpee to speak up and against studies like these and their harmful, pleasure-denying assertions.

To stimulate your or someone else's G-spot, it's helpful to remember that curvature, pressure, and positioning are your friends. Toys like the NJoy Pure Wand or a curved or bulbous-headed vibrator or dildo have the firmness, shape, and agility to stimulate this particular part of your sexual anatomy. Using plenty of lube, applying your ideal amount of pressure, and then gently rocking the toy toward the belly button (upward if you're on your back or downward if you're on hands and knees) can be a great place to start.

If using fingers, curve them using the classic come-hither motion that's become well-associated with G-spot stimulation. If an anatomical penis and/or a strap-on dildo is your chosen tool of the trade, positioning can be helpful in reaching the G-spot. Have the receiving partner tuck their knees to their chest, bend over a bed or chair, get on all fours with their chest down on the bed, or have them on top so that they can control a shallower penetration that tends to be ideal for G-spot play. Any position that essentially shortens the vaginal canal or makes penetration organically shallower or tilted toward the front of the vaginal canal is what you're shooting for here.

If you're someone who is a vaginal ejaculator, you or your partner may feel your G-spot balloon or fill with fluid! This is a great time to check in with yourself or your partner about depth, speed, and pressure and to possibly make penetration even shallower or almost outside of the body entirely to leave space for ejaculate to leave the body. Though mainstream porn may set us up to think we'll be squirting a powerful stream that'll hit the wall nine feet away from us, it's also entirely normal for ejaculate to be released from the body more like a seep, gush, or even just a gentle puddling. If you become a prolific puddle-maker, protect your mattress with some sex-designated towels or even a waterproof mattress protector.

For more extensive information on finding, stimulating, and enjoying the G-spot, here are just a few of my go-to resources:

My sex column![5] At yanatallonhicks.com, keyword search "G-spot."
The Good Vibrations Guide: The G-Spot by Cathy Winks[6] (now quite dated, but worked for me in the early 2000s!).
"My Love, The Pure Wand," an article by sex blogger Hey Epiphora at heyepiphora.com.[7]
The Secrets of Great G-Spot Orgasms and Female Ejaculation by Tristan Taormino.[8]

The most important thing I discovered that afternoon wasn't my G-spot orgasm (though that was definitely . . . *meaningful* . . . to say the least). The most valuable thing I learned was how effective and absolutely worthwhile it was to use my words during sex. With one hand holding open the book and the other playing with hook, pressure, and position, my girlfriend did her darndest to follow the halting, experimental, and at times certainly contradictory directions I was giving her—"Wait, less deep. Upward more. Maybe more pressure? Ow! No never mind go back to what you were doing before. No, not that—the other thing. Okay, wait, let's just start over. Lemme see that diagram one more time?" To an outside audience this scene might certainly not seem porn-worthy, but inside the moment, this homegrown, hands-on, G-spot educational moment felt fun, adventuresome, and like my girlfriend and I were on a quest to discover something new about my pleasure, together.

Do all successful sexual experiences need to involve a lecture and a library? No, of course not. This experience was helpful and effective for me because it helped me understand the types of stimulation that worked for my body, helped me learn how to give clearer instructions to my partner (and future partners) about this particular part of my sexual anatomy, and gave me more confidence in my body's ability to have this kind of orgasm (which—practice makes perfect!—quickly became a very reliable part of my sexual repertoire).

But what became especially clear that day is that the Classic Mood isn't necessary. So, go ahead and ruin it—kill the mood dead. What did it ever really do for you, after all, besides look good in a couple of movies a few times?

A Short Guide to Killing the Classic Mood

The good news is that killing the Classic Mood is so easy, really.

1. Prioritize yours and your partner(s)' authentic pleasure. Ask them lots of questions about what they like. Have a chat about consent, about STIs, about safety and risk, and take as much time as either of you want or need.

2. Talk during sex. About anything. Talk about what you want in the moment, what you'd like adjusted, what you might want to do next time. You could talk your dirtiest talk about all the

_____ you'd like to _____ in your partner's _____ or you could even talk clean, like about how much you like the song that's playing or how you have the same pair of underwear as your partner and you almost wore them today but then decided against it but wouldn't it have been funny and cute if you had?

3. Make adjustments to make yourself comfortable. If the blankets are uncomfortably bunched up underneath you, pause and straighten them out. If you have to pee, go to the bathroom. If the room is too hot or too cold, get up and adjust the thermostat. The Classic Mood can barely stay alive under the onslaught of your genuine physical comfort.

4. Take a break and eat a snack. One of my all-time favorite threesomes involved a long mid-sex break where we talked about politics, and comedy about politics, and ate raspberries. We laughed a lot, got our blood sugar up, and then got back to it. This would've made for really boring porn but made for a stellar real-life experience.

5. If you really want to kill that Classic Mood good and dead, get some instructional aides involved. Google something you don't know or are unsure about, preferably directly before or (dare you?) during a hook-up. Troubleshoot about how to use your fancy new vibrator and giggle as you struggle with its 100 settings and little buttons. Even read a book with real live paper pages. Bye-bye, Classic Mood—you won't be missed.

I'm not saying ALL MOODS MUST DIE. But I am saying that gathering this type of knowledge and information about my body and how it experiences pleasure would've taken a hell of a lot longer (or maybe wouldn't have happened at all) if I hadn't been able to talk about it openly, honestly, and with a big ol' question mark floating above my head during most of my attempts to figure it out—something the Classic Mood would never have condoned. Ultimately, the information we gathered during the G-spot experiments rolled over into our subtler, classically sexy, candlelit sexual experiences because (thanks to a book, our words, and sexual feedback) we now knew more about what we were doing.

Since then, my entire adult sexuality has been discovered, rediscovered, and enacted in similar ways to much success—not necessarily with an open book and an hour of dialogue every single time, but via utilizing the key pieces of this experience:

1. Knowing and giving myself permission to desire The Thing
2. Having accurate and empowering information about The Thing
3. Feeling comfortable talking to my partner about The Thing
4. Giving myself space to make mistakes, change my mind, or not know about The Thing
5. Talking about The Thing before, during, and after sex

These five crucial elements are almost always left out of the Classic Mood (especially that last one). But they're essential in creating what can grow out of the ashes of the Classic Mood: the *Authentic Mood*.

The Authentic Mood is the genuine, pleasurable, sexual space that's created by the experience of being fully ourselves in our sexual interactions. All you need to create your very own Authentic Mood is yourself, your desires, and the willingness and bravery to forge ahead without the Classic Mood's oppressive training wheels (which are mostly faulty and screwed on wrong anyway), which try to convince you that this boring cookie-cutter sex you've been having is just fine. Or maybe you're satisfied by your current sex life but want to further explore what else can be learned by continuing to peel back the layers of the sex educational onion that may be obscuring your Authentic Mood and its subsequent pleasure can bring you.

Carly and Bo started couples therapy with me for a reason many couples hire me: they weren't having as much sex as they wanted to be having. Together for three years, Carly (a graduate student) and Bo (a furniture designer) were both in their late twenties and, like many couples, had found that the spark that had had them jumping each other at every available moment in the first year of their relationship had since faded to a twice-monthly, overly familiar, routine roll in the hay. Carly's primary complaint was that she just didn't desire sex as much as she once did, and Bo felt like if it weren't for their personal individual efforts, their shared sex life would come to a complete halt.

About four sessions in, we had hit our stride in our work together, and Carly was feeling more confident in speaking about her sexual experience with Bo.

Carly: I want to want to have more sex with Bo and I want to try to initiate more but, when it crosses my mind that maybe I should start something, it just feels too hard. I'm too tired or I just don't feel up for it—I just don't feel sexy I guess.

Me: What feels difficult to you about initiating sex? [I also wanted to know what kind of sex she wants to have with Bo and if they are having it, but we'll get to this one later.]

Carly: After classes, schoolwork, dishes, and all that, I'm just too tired to be all sexy and seduce them. It just seems like so much work.

Me: Totally. Seduction takes way too much work after being in the grad-school grind, I get that.

We have a little tension-breaking chuckle and Carly looks surprised that I don't argue with her aversion to seducing her partner.

Me: Bo, do you want Carly to do a full-blown striptease for you after a long day at work?

Bo: No, not at all! I just want to like connect or have some physical affection, ya know?

Me: Okay, great. So, Carly, what would it be like if you initiated sex by saying to Bo, "I want to have sex and I'm also tired. Do you want to try to have sex and see how it goes?" Then you can get in bed together, maybe naked, with the intention of having sex, maybe you even start having sex, but also if you just end up talking about your days, eating chips, and laughing at cat memes, no big deal.

And then there's that familiar look again—do I have a dildo stuck to my face for real this time?

In Carly and Bo's case, the Classic Mood set up the expectation that to initiate sex was like getting on a rollercoaster—once you buckle yourself in, you're on the ride and there's no getting off (har har) until it's over. The Authentic Mood, on the other hand, starts with permission—permission to desire your desires, to start with where you are in the moment, and to move at your own pace, even if that pace is stop and start. The Authentic Mood is a custom job that fully embraces the energy of a perfectly imperfect sex life and sheds the illusive restraints of sexual imposter syndrome.

It was clear Carly had been internalizing her own sexual imposter syndrome by continuing to try to squish herself to fit into the Classic Mood box and giving up on sex entirely. Playing by the "rules," Carly shrunk her sexual self, unable to feel inspired to or capable of creating a customized mood box that actually, genuinely fit her and her partner. This suggestion—to clearly, and "unsexily," state your desire to have (or attempt to have) sex with your partner, with your words, in a matter-of-fact way, whilst leaving clearly delineated space for failure—is something I utilize with clients like Carly and Bo all of the time. And, nearly every time I make this suggestion, a client will start seeking a pen and paper to write it down—one of the only suggestions of mine that so consistently elicits this note-taking response.

It may seem obvious or overly simple to have to say, "Want something out of sex? Say so! Feeling a way about sex? Talk about it! Unsure how sex is going to play out today? Fess up!" In reality, the immediate and visible impact ("Huh! Do you have a pen I can borrow?") of this suggestion speaks directly to why it's such an important intervention for people to make. Our ability to take such a basic and seemingly obvious action as talking about our sex lives with the people we have sex with, openly, without the cover of metaphor, game, or mood, means that we are bucking the well-worn traditions of sex-negativity and fearmongering that have set up the Classic Mood in the first place. For this reason, actively making the shift away from the Classic Mood and toward the Authentic Mood is one that can be as challenging to initiate as it is effective. For many clients, to speak openly about their sex lives in this way is to blaze a new, unknown trail in their sexual interactions, and in the name of authentic pleasure!

6 Steps to Creating Your Own Authentic Mood

1. **Kill the Classic Mood.** Remember, ruining the Classic Mood is the easy part—talk about sex with your partner before, during, and after sex. Be yourself, where you are, in the moment that you're in right now.

2. **Practice active consent.** Active consent starts with explicit permission before any touch or sexual interaction begins, continues with checking in about how things are going, and ends with talking with each other about how the sexual interaction went overall so that feedback can be exchanged and any mistakes can be repaired (we'll get into this more in Chapter 10).

3. **Listen to your body and respond.** Your body includes your emotions, thoughts, and mental state. If something hurts, speak up and/or make adjustments. Luxuriate in your enthusiastic *yes*es, pursue physical satisfaction like you deserve it (you do!), and remember that you get to decide what feels good to you and your body.

4. Practice bravery in asking for what you want (Chapter 7 is *all* about this!). Offer instruction, constructive editing, and enthusiastic agreement about whether or not your partner is understanding what you're asking for. Create a sex life where you and your partner feel more empowered and able to speak up if something isn't working and are less likely to agree to something you're/they're not enthusiastic about (see Chapter 11).

5. Connect with what genuinely makes you feel sexy, and accept what those components are, without worrying about whether or not your sexy is everyone's sexy (statistically, an impossibility). Context matters when it comes to feeling your sexiest, so pay attention to the details and/or start taking note of what makes your brain and body feel good both inside and out of explicit sexual contexts.

6. The Authentic Mood isn't just about what you want, it's also about what your partner wants and where the two of you intersect. You and your partner(s) may be super into certain acts, kinks, or interests, and in some situations, one of you may be fiery hot for something while the other is lukewarm. You don't need to agree on every single aspect of what constitutes your ideal Authentic Mood in order to create one between the two (or more) of you (see Chapter 11). Start with taking a nonjudgmental stance about your partner's desires to begin creating a safer space to talk about what each of you really want.

Does this list feel impossible to check off or even get started on? You're not alone. Oftentimes clients will leave my office thoroughly convinced that creating an Authentic Mood is a great idea! And then they'll come back the next week with a new barrier: "I want to state my actual needs, wants, and desires to my partner before, during, and after sex, I really do—but I honestly don't even know what those desires are." For many people, the feeling or realization that you might not truly know what you want or what brings you pleasure can be curious, disappointing, or downright distressing.

Particularly for queer folks and/or women, it can tend toward the latter, as depriving ourselves of pleasure has been made a structurally enforced, oppressive social norm—don't dress or look like this, don't eat that, don't lust, don't want, don't achieve too much but also never fail. Simply knowing what brings you genuine pleasure can be a groundbreaking, radical, and sometimes thigh-trembling place of power. Before we can know exactly what we want, we've got to give ourselves permission to want in the first place. The Authentic Mood can grant us just that.

Creating the Authentic Mood isn't just an issue of opening space for more pleasurable sex but a crucial component to creating more consensual, more empowered, and more identity-enriching experiences of our bodies, our personhood, and how we relate to intimacy, connection, and others. No. Big. Deal.

Ding-dong, the Classic Mood is dead.

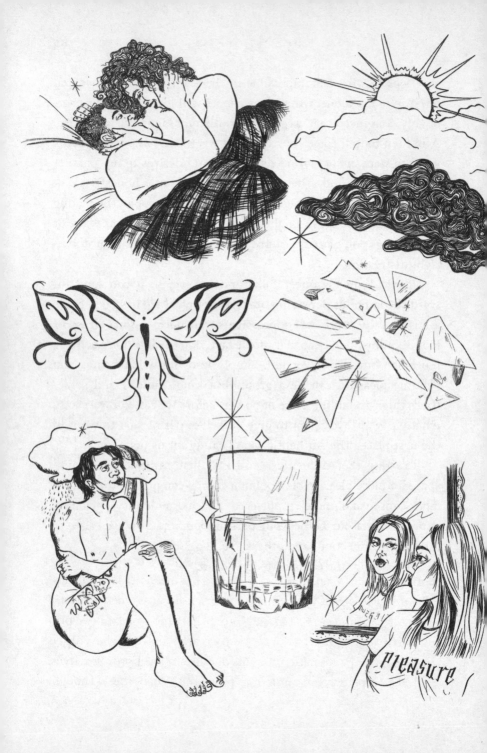

CHAPTER 4

Barrier #2: Pleasure Pessimism

No problem can be solved from the same
level of consciousness that created it.[1]
—Albert Einstein

This is why we can't have nice things.[2]
—Paula Poundstone

The Authentic Mood requires your full participation in creating it: asking for what you want (Chapter 7), giving yourself permission to desire (Chapter 6), and identifying your boundaries (Chapter 8)—none of which can happen without a fundamental frame of mind that says, "Yes! Authentic pleasure can happen here!" Or, at the very least, it takes an ongoing commitment to work toward cultivating a frame of mind that believes in your own authentic pleasure potential.

Unfortunately, most of us are steeped in negative or conflicting messages about sex for so long that they become an almost unnoticeable backdrop to our sex lives. This means that regardless of our best sex-positive efforts, these sex-negative messages still easily sneak under the radar of our beliefs (no matter how pro-pleasure, feminist, or sex educated we are!) and can show up as barely noticed automatic thoughts about ourselves, our sex lives, and our capacity for authentic pleasure. When these thought loops snowball, they create an interlocking network of unhelpful beliefs, feelings, and behaviors in our sex lives, forming a neat little pleasure-limiting package I like to call *Pleasure Pessimism*.

Pleasure Pessimism starts with an unhelpful belief about your sexual self, your partner(s), and your sex life. This belief is then compounded and supported by automatic thoughts that discourage you from pursuing your authentic pleasure and desires during sex. Automatic thoughts are thoughts that occur so frequently that they usually go unnoticed. In your sex life, pleasure-pessimistic automatic thoughts act as small-but-mighty barricades that stop you from taking the actions necessary to create the sex life you actually want. Automatic thoughts on their own are usually no big deal but, repeated and diversified enough, they can easily form and/or support a cumulative, counterproductive belief that can be taken for granted as the truth and therefore slide by unnoticed and unchallenged.

A common example of this pattern is one I hear typically from people with vulvas: "I take too long to climax." This belief is often rooted in and reinforced by several automatic thoughts that might occur throughout a sexual interaction: "My partner must be bored," "Her jaw probably hurts by now," "Ugh, I'm taking FOREVER to come," "Why am I taking so long?", "C'mon body, hurry up and climax already!" Because of this (unhelpful, unverified, and unvoiced) thought and belief network, this person might modify their sexual behavior to account for it: they might not ask for cunnilingus at all even though they love it, they might cut a sex act shorter than they (or maybe even their partner) would like, they might have a hard time feeling pleasure or climaxing because of their resulting "hurry up" anxiety, or they might even fake an orgasm to rid themselves of said anxiety.

These automatic thoughts don't come out of nowhere and are born out of sex-negative contextual factors such as media, sex education, cultural shame, and sexual misinformation. (Don't forget! It takes the average person with a vulva 14 minutes of direct, consistent clitoral stimulation in order to climax[3] and most do not routinely, and some never, experience orgasm solely from sexual intercourse.[4])

Sometimes, our automatic thoughts are repeatedly reinforced through real-life experiences such as unsatisfying sexual encounters, failed attempts at talking to your partner(s) about sex, or being outright shamed for your sexual desires or habits.[5] When our negative thoughts about our sexuality are reinforced in this way, our unhelpful beliefs can concretize even further: "I take too long to climax from cunnilingus, which bores my partner" (as "proven" by the one partner I had who once said they were bored during cunnilingus because I was taking too long). We then naturally attempt to protect ourselves from continued sexual shame, discomfort, or awkwardness by modifying our behavior in a preventative way ("I won't ask for cunnilingus from any other partners ever again" or "It's already been ten minutes, I'll initiate a shift in sexual activity now to prevent boredom for my partner"). It would be understandable that a person with this particular network of automatic thoughts, beliefs, behaviors, and sexual experiences might enter a sexual encounter feeling rushed, anxious, defeated, or otherwise not present in the sex they're having. This person might also communicate less, shy away from asking for what they want, or be distracted in engaging with their partner's desires and boundaries.

The ripple effect of automatic thoughts, beliefs, behaviors, and feelings has been heavily studied by a facet of talk therapy called cognitive behavioral therapy (CBT),[6] which was described in Chapter 3. CBT is a form of evidence-based therapy that guides clients through identifying, unraveling, and reorganizing their thoughts, beliefs, and behaviors pertaining to a particularly distressing topic. CBT works to shift a client's core narrative about the particularly distressing topic from one of limiting negativity ("I take too long to climax") to one of hopeful flexibility ("Everyone's climax time varies and so does mine. As long as my partner and I are both enjoying what we're doing and check in about it, there's no such thing as taking too long"). CBT has been proven to be especially effective for folks battling anxiety, depression, and phobias[7] and is an approach I use often with clients who are struggling with pleasure-pessimistic thought/behavior patterns about sex. Pleasure-pessimistic belief systems are often triggered by unhelpful thoughts about sex, ourselves, or our partners that then set off a domino effect of self-sabotaging actions and unsatisfying sexual experiences. In this chapter, you'll explore your own unique Pleasure Pessimism through identifying your particular network of unhelpful thoughts and beliefs, and the ripple effect they set off in your sex life. In the next chapter, we'll be using CBT strategies to untangle and recreate your resulting Negative Narratives to cultivate more positive and pleasure-centered thoughts and behaviors in their place.

Unhelpful Automatic Thoughts and Messages

Before I sat down to write this chapter, I crowdsourced some examples of Pleasure Pessimism on my Instagram account. I posted a story with a question box that asked, "What are the unhelpful things you tell yourself that have blocked (or still block) you from asking for what you want out of sex?" The responses I received are listed below and echo sentiments I frequently hear from my clients, sex column readers, peers, and even (yes, sometimes still) from within myself. You'll find the responses broken into three categories: learned lies, negative stories I fear repeating, and beliefs about myself and/or my partner(s). Of course, these categories are not cleanly cut from each other and often overlap, so feel free to consider what other category each response might fit in. You might notice when reading these lists that some of these statements resonate more strongly with your own personal experience than others. I encourage you to circle or make a note by the ones that stand out.

Learned Lies

Learned lies is a category that describes thoughts or beliefs that are based on a stereotype, myth, generalization, or otherwise untrue "fact" about sex, pleasure, and sexuality. These lies are learned either overtly from sex education (formal or at-home) or covertly from media, social interactions, and what is considered taboo or "normal." For example, as you see in the first response listed, "She'll think I'm 'too gay'" is an often homophobia-laden thought based on the idea that certain sex acts are only acted on or enjoyed by gay men (i.e., anal sex, prostate stimulation), which is not true. Learned lies include assumptions like:

- She'll think I'm "too gay."
- They'll think I'm "too straight."
- My pleasure deserves less attention because my libido is · lower.

- Asking for something kinky from someone less kinky than you is asking too much.
- Fat girls should be thankful for any attention at all.
- Meeting my partner's needs is the priority; meeting my own needs is not.
- I should hold back my pleasure response in case it's not "sexy" to my partner.
- I enjoy multiple orgasms, which is too much to ask for; I should be satisfied with one and get over it.
- I shouldn't ask too much, especially if I'm kinkier than my partner.
- I should always get off—so I make moaning noises that are over-the-top and not organic.
- It's too much of a hassle to ask for XYZ.
- He should already know what I want.
- Good girls don't ask.
- My partner's pleasure matters more than mine (a good lover is entirely other-focused).
- Nobody wants to hear about how I'm triggered.
- It feels rude to ask for what I want.
- I'm being selfish if I ask for what I want.

Negative Stories I Fear Repeating

This category includes thoughts and beliefs that have often been reinforced by a real-life experience or were created by a real-life experience. The automatic thoughts connected to negative stories often include the fear that this real-life experience will repeat and are unconsciously created in the hopes of preventing this repetition.

- It's always been hard for me to come and I worry that partners will get annoyed or bored.
- What if they don't want or like it that way?
- It's going to take too much time.
- It's too effortful for them.
- It's not fun to be the director of the sexual experience; I want my partner to take on that role.
- I'm afraid and embarrassed that I'll be rejected, invalidated, or humiliated.
- What if what I want makes their body uncomfortable (for example, hurts their jaw if they go down on me for too long)?
- I've asked for what I want before without any positive impact so why should I ask again?
- I don't ask in casual sex situations because of the extra emotional labor of explaining what I want and trying to get it right   it's not worth it.

Beliefs about Myself and/or My Partner(s)

Beliefs are some of the hardest sex-negative messages to resist because they have been so clearly labeled as "the truth" in our minds for so long that we rarely consider or try out alternatives to them. Beliefs are often expressed as assumptions and are thought to be universal or unchangeable (though, thankfully, many of them are not!). Usually, they are accompanied by the ultimate fear of rejection.

- If my partner were interested in that thing, they'd do it more already or initiate it, and because they haven't they must not be into it so I shouldn't ask.

- I'm happy with what we normally do. I don't *need* anything beyond that even though I *want* something beyond that.
- I don't know what I want; I've always been focused on the other person.
- This will sound dumb if I say it out loud.
- I fear she only experiments to please me, not because she is as curious as I am to explore.
- I don't deserve to feel good.
- My partner's pleasure should always be more important than mine.
- It must annoy my partner when I ask for things.
- My parts are unattractive so I have to have the lights off or the blankets on during sex.
- They're only doing this because I asked them to do it, which means they don't actually like it.
- I'm too old to experiment with my sexuality at this point.
- "People like me" don't do kink.
- I don't know what I want and I don't know how to find out.
- I don't like that thing (even though I've never even allowed myself to try it so how would I know?).

Automatic thoughts can feel like a cognitive tug-of-war between your larger sexual values and the quick thoughts that pop into your head about or during sex. This can make them harder to catch (and therefore harder to change). Shining a light of awareness on your automatic thoughts can help you expose their impact on your sex life and identify your own Pleasure Pessimism, which we'll do in the following exercise. If this exercise has you drawing blanks, make it your next self-experiment to try to catch or notice your automatic thoughts next time you're masturbating, with your sexual partner, or when you're fantasizing about your next sexual experience. You can even make this a collaborative project with a current partner and let them in on your self-assigned homework, inviting them to join in on their own self-noticing. This may even have the added benefit of building more transparency and intimacy into your sex life.

Brainstorm Box #1: My Unhelpful Automatic Thoughts

Your turn! Jot down some of the unhelpful thoughts or beliefs you have about yourself, your sex life, and/or your partner(s) that block you from asking for what you really want out of sex. You're welcome to categorize them or use my categories (learned lies, negative stories I fear repeating, beliefs about myself and/or my partner[s]) as brainstorming prompts, or you can just write your list free-form.

What are the unhelpful messages you tell yourself that have blocked (or still block) you from asking for what you want out of sex?

_____

_____

_____

_____

_____

_____

_____

It's important to recognize that, although your automatic thoughts and Pleasure Pessimism are unique to you, they are not your fault. Our sex lives and how we feel about them are not individual nor simple projects. We as a human species in general have really messed up our approach to this whole sex thing. We have to turn inward to look at our own pleasure-pessimistic thought patterns as individuals, but it's important to not let the larger forces at work off the hook of responsibility. In my casual Instagram "research," I encouraged people to zoom out a little by posting this follow-up question: "Where do you think you learned these unhelpful messages?" Below are the responses I received:

- Media and peers
- Home
- The message that penis-in-vagina sex is the only definition of/way to have sex
- Religion/church
- Men telling me that they didn't like certain acts when actually they just didn't want to "have to" do them or work to pleasure me
- A lack of sex education or safe sources to ask about sex
- Being socialized to make every situation comfortable for the other person
- Viewing media where sex is portrayed as "just feeling good" automatically, without conversation
- My experience of being with guys who didn't care about my pleasure
- Patriarchy
- General kink-shaming that I've internalized
- *Gestures widely at the socialization I've experienced being a woman of color*

- Movies, TV, mainstream ideals of porn, American puritanical culture
- Porn, society, ex-partners
- Fetishism pertaining to racial stereotypes applied to my body

---

Brainstorm Box #2: Where Do You Think You Learned These Unhelpful Messages?

Your turn! Some of our unhelpful messages and thought patterns can be influenced by several sources or experiences that converge into a deeply rooted belief or fear. It can also be tricky to accurately pinpoint the influences on your own automatic thoughts (sometimes working with a therapist can be helpful here!). Let's give it a shot anyway. Return to your list of unhelpful messages from the box above and write down the influencing "truths," sources, and entities in your life you think may have played a role in shaping them.

_____

_____

_____

_____

_____

_____

_____

_____

Though these larger contextual factors are often not within your control to change (at least not immediately nor completely), addressing the roots, triggers, and ripple effect of your own unique Pleasure Pessimism *is in your power* and is also a worthy endeavor. By doing so, you can identify what your specific automatic, pleasure-blocking thoughts are, actively resist the wider sex-negative contextual influences that have informed them, and shine a light on your previously unchecked pessimistic beliefs. Ultimately, this will reduce Pleasure Pessimism's presence in and power over your sex life, and open pathways to easier sexual communication, higher sexual self-esteem, and more pleasure-packed sexual encounters.

Jessa and Levi
Pleasure Pessimism at Play

Jessa is a recent college graduate now working in college admissions. She is self-identified as an "anxious person in general" and openly discusses how anxiety can hijack her sexual experiences with Levi, her partner of three years. She says that they've always had a somewhat stunted sex life and heavily blames her own anxiety for this. She describes a sex life where at least one anxiety hurdle needs to be cleared every time they have sex (What if I don't get off? What if I change my mind midway through sex? What if I don't like what we're doing?) and even during (Why isn't he changing positions? I wish he would touch my clitoris more. I wonder if the noises I'm making are too weird or loud. I want to ask for my vibrator but don't want to hurt his feelings.). When she lands in my office,

Jessa is starting to lose all hope that she and Levi will ever share a satisfying sex life—she's fed up and frustrated that he "just doesn't get me" and isn't giving her the kind of sexual experience she wants to have as a "young, feminist, sex-positive woman who just wants to be having good sex already."

In our subsequent exploration of her sexual stories, I sense a heaping spoonful of Pleasure Pessimism is in the mix here. I test my theory by asking Jessa a couple of questions. When I ask her, "How does Levi respond when you tell him how you want to be touched?" she says she doesn't give him much direction, and when I ask, "Do you think he's listening to your feedback?" she says she gives him bodily clues or changes the noises she's making and that "he's just not paying attention." It turns out Jessa has never directly said, "Not like that, like this" or "I'd love to see XYZ go differently next time" or even "You know what I would really love is . . ." This doesn't mean that this unsatisfying sexual dynamic is Jessa's *fault*, and it doesn't mean that Levi couldn't sharpen his own sexual communication skills, but it does point to some barriers in the forms of automatic thoughts and unhelpful beliefs. This is what I was interested in highlighting for Jessa.

"What do you think is stopping you from letting Levi know, clearly and verbally, what you want out of the sex you're having?" I ask her. I've asked this question of many clients in many ways. Typical responses I've gotten more than once are "I don't know what I want," "I don't want to be embarrassed," "I don't want to ruin the mood." Jessa gives me an answer that I think people rarely say aloud but often believe without thinking much about it: "I just want him to know how to have sex with me."

The desire for our partners to read our minds is organic, common, and, quite frankly, relatable. We want to be seen and known by our partners. We want them to have paid enough attention to our needs and desires to be able to predict our future wants. Our (sometimes unreasonable) inner child may even want our mind-melding to be powerful enough to heal our past relational wounds inflicted by years of not feeling heard, seen, or like we mattered. Perhaps most importantly in the realm of sex, we don't want to have to take the vulnerable risk of saying "I want" or face possible rejection from the people we care about the most when we ask, "Can I have?" If partners could read each other's minds I might very well be put out of business but alas, here we are, needing to practice our direct communication skills instead.

"Have you ever directly and verbally told Levi how you want him to have sex with you?" I ask Jessa.

"I guess not *directly*," she answers.

"Well then, how is he supposed to know?" I joke lightly.

After some discussion about whether or not Jessa's largely nonverbal communication attempts have been effective (they have not), Jessa comes to the conclusion that there might be some other ways to navigate this sexual conundrum besides waiting for Levi to guess correctly or just giving up on their sexual relationship entirely. I can't help but agree.

It seems simple enough to say, "If you want him to know the thing, tell him the thing," but of course, it's not. Jessa's own network of Pleasure Pessimism has solidified the unhelpful belief that Levi should *know* what to do, which then cascades into a litany of automatic thoughts about Levi's very human lack of mind-reading capabilities ("Why isn't he touching me the way I want to be touched?", "He doesn't care about my pleasure," "He's clearly not into this") and Jessa's own options for how to proceed ("It's too late to talk about this now," "I don't know how to describe what I want," "I shouldn't have to give him directions").

Though Levi himself is not in the therapy room, it's also likely that he, too, believes that he should "just know how to have sex with my girlfriend" without having much guidance around how to do that or any examples of how to ask someone what it is they want out of sex, how to ask for and accept feedback (Chapter 9), or how to co-create a sexual experience with another person. When belief systems like this overlap in a relationship they're harder to notice or challenge because both people are taking that belief for granted. As a result, partners can get stalled out and frustrated as they attempt to work *around* this unhelpful belief rather than critically examine whether or not this belief is *actually working for them* and, if not, what to do about it.

Luckily, it only takes one person to shift a dynamic pattern, and today that person is Jessa. We start by drawing a map of influences around Jessa's pleasure-pessimistic belief that "He should just know what I want out of sex." By asking questions like, "How did you learn that your partner should just know what you want without being told?", "What experiences have you had that back up that belief?", and "What else have you learned about sex and relationships that influence this belief?", Jessa and I draw out the following visual map of other thoughts, experiences, beliefs, and feelings that have played a role here such as her own fear of asking for what she wants, her socially enforced idea that men should be in charge of sexual interactions, and that it's her job as a "good sex partner" to not offend Levi's ego by offering suggestions or direction during sex.

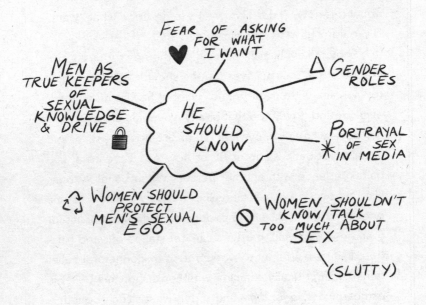

FEAR OF ASKING FOR WHAT I WANT

MEN AS TRUE KEEPERS OF SEXUAL KNOWLEDGE & DRIVE

△ GENDER ROLES

HE SHOULD KNOW

PORTRAYAL * OF SEX IN MEDIA

WOMEN SHOULD PROTECT MEN'S SEXUAL EGO

WOMEN SHOULDN'T KNOW/TALK TOO MUCH ABOUT SEX

(SLUTTY)

My Map of Pleasure-Pessimistic Influences

Your turn! Choose one unhelpful automatic thought from Brainstorm Box #1 on page 95. Write it in the center circle. Then, write down the various influences, companion messages, experiences, and other beliefs you might hold that unhelpfully reinforce this automatic thought or belief. If you're feeling stuck, refer to your answers to Brainstorm Box #2 on page 97 for examples of outside influences.

Pro tip: this is a simple map to draw out in a separate journal or piece of paper. You might like to do this exercise more than once.

*My MAP OF *
PLEASURE -,PESSIMISM

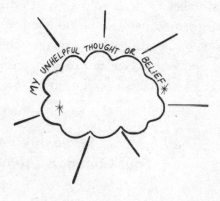

Acknowledging what's influencing our Pleasure Pessimism, whether visually like in the map above, written in a list form in your journal, or talked about over tea with your partner, does what us therapists like to call *externalizing the problem* (a concept we'll get into more in Chapter 11). When we acknowledge the external forces that are supporting our problems we can say "something's not quite right here" rather than situating blame as "something's wrong with my partner" or "something's wrong with me." Not only are the latter two thoughts damaging to your self-esteem, your relational connection, and your sex life, but they also create an understanding of the problem as an unchangeable truth rather than as a workable challenge. When we can visualize a big portion of the problem as being caused by the context rather than caused by a particular person, we're less likely to believe "I'm broken" or "My partner's broken," which only serves to drive a wedge between you, your partner, and your pleasure rather than inspiring you to say, "Dang, society really fucked up this whole sex thing. Let's see what we can do to overcome Pleasure Pessimism and create a sex life that is free to flourish despite our sex-negative world."

The Impacts of Pleasure Pessimism (Four Common Themes)

The beliefs and automatic thoughts that we hold about sex and sexuality impact how we show up to our real, everyday (well, maybe not *every*day) sex lives. The research behind CBT[8] has shown the mental health community that thoughts and beliefs absolutely influence our emotions, actions, and behaviors. If you change one, you change the patterned way they are all linked together. When we can identify our pleasure-pessimistic automatic thoughts and beliefs, we can then look at how the way we've been *thinking* about our sex lives has directly influenced that way we *feel* and *act* during sex, in our relationships, or in regard to our sex lives as a whole.

When we are operating from a place of Pleasure Pessimism, we are more likely to feel negatively about our sexual selves, our partners, and our potential for sexual pleasure. We are also more likely to behave in a way that supports that pessimistic belief system: shutting down, staying quiet, refraining from sharing desires, being overly porous or rigid with our boundaries, avoiding sex all together, or otherwise communicating in a lackluster way about our sexual experience. If we are able to shift our patterns toward Pleasure Optimism instead, we may be able to interrupt this cycle enough times to create a new understanding of our sex lives as a place of satisfaction, pleasure, successful communication, and possibility, with the pleasure-positive thoughts, feelings, beliefs, and behaviors to back it up. In order to get there, however, we've got to understand the current way our Pleasure Pessimism has been impacting our feelings and behaviors up until this point.

Everyone's Pleasure Pessimism is unique because our automatic thoughts and behaviors have been influenced by our individual experiences, our various identities, and the cultural contexts that we have been raised in and live in. However, because sex has been negatively impacted by some general messages, there are common pleasure-pessimistic themes I've noticed in my last decade-plus of being a sex educator. Below, I detail four of them, identifying for each an automatic thought that might accompany it, the feelings it may cause, the behaviors it may result in, and the overall impact it might have on a person's sex life. As you read these, take note of any themes that stand out to you in your own sexual experience.

1. The Goldilocks Effect: How much pleasure you experience from sex and how you display that pleasure (i.e., via erections, wetness, orgasms, noise-making, etc.) needs to be just right. There is both a cap on having/displaying *too much* pleasure but also a bottom line of having/displaying *not enough* pleasure. (Seems like a trap, right? Probably because it is). Rather than being present for your real sexual experience, this mode of thinking has people caught up in worrying about how their partner is perceiving them and what the performance of their pleasure should look like, moving them further away from authentic pleasure and sexual satisfaction.

   Theme: I'm too much/not enough.

   Thoughts: "This vibrator she's using on me feels great but I'm taking forever to climax today for some reason! I should've climaxed by now for sure. She must be getting impatient. What if she thinks I don't like it?"

   Feelings: Anxiety, rushed, worried.

   Behaviors: Less likely to climax because of those feelings, prematurely ends vibrator time she was totally enjoying without saying anything to her partner about it.

   Impact: Cuts herself off from pleasure because she wasn't getting "results" fast enough.

2. No, I Insist, After You: Most people feel hesitant to ask for what they want out of sex, but they also simultaneously report a genuine desire to know what their partners want. Clients often tell me that they feel nervous, shy, or overly vulnerable in asking for what they want out of sex or they fear being perceived as demanding, as a burden,

as a creep, or as "too slutty" if they do eventually ask (we'll cover the art of asking in Chapter 7).

The interesting part here is that most people don't apply these same rules to their *partners* asking for *their* sexual wants. Rather than assume that their partner might also have these hang-ups, people often think, "Certainly, my partner would just freely share any desires they might have, so if they're not asking for something they must not be interested in it!" As a result, people refrain from sharing their own sexual wants while simultaneously taking their partners' lack of forthrightness as confirmation of their lack of interest in a particular sex act, dynamic, or desire.

If this is the stance everyone in a given sexual encounter is taking, holding the door open for each other forever, then nobody ever walks through it and we're all just stuck standing there, waiting for something to happen and wondering why we're not getting what we want out of sex.

Theme: I'll wait for my partner to bring up this desire I have instead of asking for it directly myself.

Thoughts: "I want to try this new kinky thing but my partner hasn't ever mentioned it to me, so he's not into it. I shouldn't even bring it up because he'll probably feel like I'm pressuring him to do something he doesn't want to do."

Feelings: Self-doubt, disconnect from partner, like a kinky weirdo, sexually stifled, unsatisfied.

Behaviors: Never brings it up based on the assumption that his partner isn't into it.

Impacts: Doesn't give his partner the opportunity to explore kink with him. Doesn't give his partner the opportunity to set his own boundaries nor is this person displaying trust in his partner's ability to say no or yes. Never finds out or gives his partner the chance to share his own thoughts, feelings, and desires about that kink. Eventually feels trapped and forced to choose between his current partner and their current sex life or a new, kink-inclusive sex life with somebody else.

3.   People Pleasing (Literally): This one often goes along with #2 but is more specifically geared toward the belief that your partner(s)' pleasure matters more than yours and should always be the focus no matter what. This theme is complex because it is often born out of modern consent culture and sex positivity, which rightfully encourages people to be mindful of other people's boundaries, desires, and sexual satisfaction.

However, if this other-focus becomes the *only* focus, this mode of thinking can lead to people staying quiet about their *own* desires, needs, and boundaries and/or discouraging themselves from luxuriating for "too long" in their own pleasurable experience (oral sex, anyone?). Again, if everyone in a given sexual encounter is taking this stance, when does enjoying pleasure get to happen?

Theme: My partner's pleasure is always the priority over mine.

Thoughts: "A good sexual partner is a good sexual host, so I should put my partner's sexual goals above my own at all times."

Feelings: Disconnected from their sexual self, unsure of their own wants, cloudy about their boundaries.

Behaviors: Always puts their partners in the sexual driver's seat and rarely ever explores their own pleasure; creates one-sided sexual interactions that don't feel entirely satisfying or collaborative to either person in the room.

Impacts: Gets really good at pleasing others and derives sexual self-esteem from doing so. However, is totally stumped when a partner eventually asks them what *they* want and then feels inadequate, confused, and sexually immature because they have no idea how to answer that question or advocate for their own pleasure.

4. Hook, Line, and (Pleasure) Sinker: This Pleasure Pessimism theme can be summarized as follows: "I've bought the mass-enforced lie [insert sexual untruth here] for so long that I haven't stopped to question it or to ask my partner what their stance on the issue is." As a result, people act first in response to this misinformed belief rather than stopping to think critically about this belief and whether or not it actually serves them, holds true for them, or influences the way their partner views sex.

This theme is very present in Jessa's dilemma and in her map of influences. To use an additional example, "Straight men don't enjoy anal sex" is a commonly held belief and commonly repeated myth. It's also not true and has been heavily influenced by homophobia, transphobia, and misinformation about sexual pleasure. Rather than considering an alternative to this belief or talking to his partner about whether or not they're actually interested in anal sex, a straight, cisgender man who has internalized this sexual untruth might avoid bringing up his interest in receiving anal sex or might dampen his authentic pleasure response if/when he does try receiving it, all based on the assumption that "Straight men don't enjoy anal sex" is *the truth*.

Theme: [Insert sexual untruth here] is *the truth* and I'm an outlier who needs to get back in line.

Thoughts: "I'm super interested in exploring receiving anal sex and it turns me on to fantasize about it but straight men don't enjoy anal sex and I'm not gay so . . ."

Feelings: Confused about his sexuality, ashamed of his sexual desires, nervous about being found out by his partner, but still curious about receiving anal sex!

Behaviors: Shuts down conversations about new sexual desires with his girlfriend, avoids his booty like a hot stove, continues to feel confused and guilty when he fantasizes about it.

Impacts: Never has the opportunity to challenge this belief via reading about anal sex, talking to other straight dudes who enjoy receiving anal, or creating an open environment where he and his girlfriend could experience this new thing together. Never knows if maybe his girlfriend is indeed into this.

When we are able to lay out the domino effect of pleasure-pessimistic thoughts, beliefs, feelings, behaviors, and impacts, we begin to have a clearer idea of where we can break and then redirect the cycle of Pleasure Pessimism. You can chart out your own personal cycle of Pleasure Pessimism by looking at the ways your own pleasure-pessimistic thoughts impact your feelings and behaviors in your sex life, starting with the worksheet below.

My Pleasure-Pessimism Cycle

Return to your answers to Brainstorm Box #1 (page 95) about unhelpful automatic thoughts. Choose one to focus on here to begin exploring the way this thought impacts your emotions, behaviors, and beliefs about your sex life.

My Unhelpful Automatic Thought:

Jessa's example: Levi should just know how to have sex with me.

Feelings/Emotions: What do I feel what I think this thought?

Jessa's example: Disempowered, annoyed, frustrated, uncared for, unnoticed

Behaviors/Actions: What do I do or not do in my sex life when I think this thought?

Jessa's example: I expect Levi to read my mind. I don't ask for what I want from sex. I don't explore what I want out of sex. I leave Levi completely in charge of my sexual satisfaction.

Impacts: How does this pattern barricade me from genuine sexual pleasure?

Jessa's example: I don't give Levi the opportunity to learn more about me or know me deeply as a sexual person. I set up a pattern of not offering corrections or feedback, which is then a pattern that is hard to break. I don't have as much fun as I could be having! I blame Levi if the sex we have doesn't feel good.

Impacts/Secondary Gains: How does this pattern benefit me?

(Note: This can be a tricky question. Many of our problematic thought/behavior patterns are kept in place by some of the unseen or coincidental benefits they provide us [called *secondary gains*[9] in traditional psychology]. If we can acknowledge these coincidental benefits, it can be possible to find ways to seek these benefits elsewhere or decrease our reliance on them rather than continuing our problematic pattern in order to keep those benefits in place).

Jessa's example: If I leave Levi in charge, I don't have to be vulnerable and ask for what I want or share my desires. If Levi guesses what I want correctly, I can get that "take me now!" or mind-melding feeling I love so much. I feel confident that I'm supporting Levi's sexual confidence, ego, and masculinity if I continue to let him be in charge or provide the illusion that I'm satisfied with everything he does.

By illustrating and exploring her sexual issues with Levi in these ways (first, by mapping out the contextual influences of the problem, and then, by parsing out her thought-feeling-belief-behavior cycle), Jessa is able to see the full picture of her own unique Pleasure Pessimism. Rather than get caught up in the ineffective habit of either blaming her partner or blaming herself, Jessa has zoomed out her lens to include the many other factors that contribute to her current sexual dissatisfaction. She is also now free to take a more empowered stance in contributing to changing these pleasure-pessimistic patterns because she better understands how her own way of thinking about her sex life, herself, and her partner has been keeping her stuck in this sexual rut.

Luckily for Jessa and for us all, Pleasure Pessimism is not a permanent part of *you* or *who you are*. It is a changeable belief system made up of a well-worn pattern of thoughts, feelings, and actions. Meaning: we can modify our relationship to our own pleasure-pessimistic thoughts and behaviors in order to greatly diminish their impact on our sexual experiences, our relationships, and on our ability to communicate about our sexual needs, wants, and desires.

In the next chapter, we'll explore how to do just this. Like Jessa, we all have options when it comes to shifting our cognitive orientation to our own sexual pleasure from one of automatic, unnoticed pessimism to intentional, ever-evolving Pleasure Optimism. We can learn to think about our pleasure differently, we can take action that breaks the cycle of Pleasure Pessimism in our sex lives, or we can do both. According to CBT, if you think and act differently, you'll feel and experience differently. Or, in this case, you'll change the way you think about and prioritize pleasure, and create new, more pleasurable experiences in your sex life.

Pleasure Pep Talk!

Before we move on, let's do a quick, motivational check-in.

1. **If you could reduce the power Pleasure Pessimism has over your sex life, how do you think it would positively impact your sexual experiences, relationships, or sexual self-esteem?**

Be specific. Try the prompt, "Instead of doing/feeling/ thinking _____, I would be doing/feeling/thinking _____."

2. **Do you think it's possible for you to change your pleasure-pessimistic beliefs and reduce the frequency of your pleasure-pessimistic thoughts, behaviors, and feelings?**

(Psst, I do. Because that's what we're about to do next!) If not, make a quick list of what you think still stands in your way.

Orgasms Aren't Faked for No Dang Reason!

"Stop faking orgasms!" We've all seen this well-intentioned battle cry on the sex-positive internet. However, many fail to consider the contributing factors that lead to a faked orgasm in the first place. Instead, we turn to blaming the would-be-orgasm-haver for faking it as we demand that they simply do things differently. However, orgasms don't just fake themselves nor is the pattern of faking climax one that developed on its own, in a vacuum. If we really want to stop this pleasure-sabotaging, fake-it phenomenon, we need to first acknowledge the wider forces that have influenced the great fake and what we can *all* do to reverse this course besides simply yelling, "Stop faking!" into the digital void.

A person may feel inclined to fake their pleasure for several reasons:

- Not having had the pleasure-focused sex education to know how to experience an orgasm at all or specifically how to do this with a partner.

- Wanting the sexual interaction to end and not feeling safe or confident enough to end it in another way.

- Shame around not being able to climax or fearing that they're "taking too long" and not wanting to share this information with their partner.

- Fear of revealing an underlying cause of orgasm difficulties such as trauma, medication, injury, or disability.

- Feeling embarrassed or unable to tell their partner directly what they know helps them climax.

- Fear and avoidance of hurting a partner's feelings or sexual ego.

- Widespread histories of gendered, sexual, and racial violence that can discourage people (particularly women and queer people) from speaking up to a partner about what they do not like or want from them sexually.

So, what are some ways that you can be proactive in making space for your partner's genuine pleasure?

- Deprioritize orgasm as the goal of sex. Lowered pressure to climax can often lead to more pleasure, organically. When the goal isn't climax, other things are free to happen without anyone rushing or feeling like a failure.

- Ask your partner what they want out of sex and check in often about how things are feeling.

- Listen to their suggestions and feedback without getting tripped up by your own ego (much more on this in Chapter 9).

- Speak up about your own needs and experience of pleasure during sex. You can set the tone of honest and open communication in your sexual interactions and model how this kind of communication might go.

- Ask your partner for their thoughts and ideas about what

to do during sex; they know their sexual body and desires way more than you do so treat them like the expert they are. Don't forget to continue these conversations after sex as well as outside of actively sexual moments.

- Work to create sexual safety for *everyone*—in your personal life, your sexual life, and in the world at large.

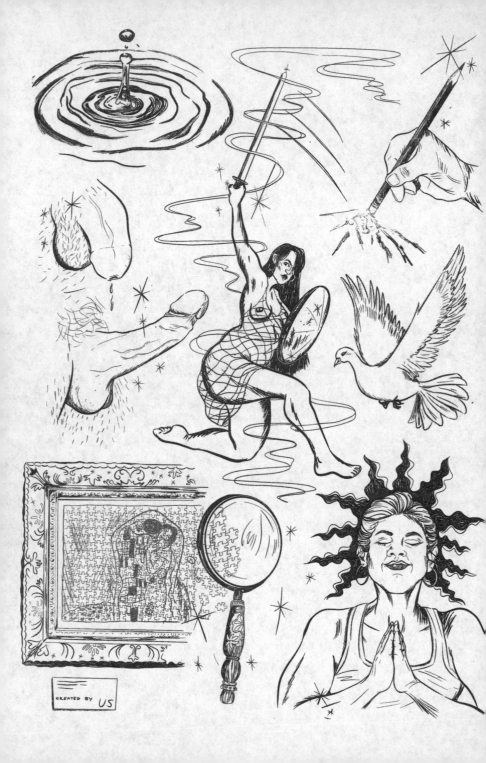

CREATED BY US

CHAPTER 5

Reshaping Negative Narratives

*You're going to tell yourself stories anyway, so
why not tell yourself the good ones?*[1]
—Jodie Rogers, empowerment coach and speaker

"Erections are super emotional," I tell my new couple client midway through their first session. I pause for a beat, waiting to see if I've just entirely lost Clark and Maria to this (admittedly) impulsive phrasing. They've just finished telling me the story of the sexual problem that has brought them to therapy. They look back at me, I assume waiting for more, so I try for a more professional tone, adding, "It's important that we acknowledge that erections are both hypervisible in a sexual interaction and also require safety and care in order to be present."

To my own relief and surprise (though, let's be honest, being surprised by anyone after ten years of fielding sexual quandaries should really be out of my system by now), Clark nods thoughtfully, seemingly taking in my point of view. Clark owns a small factory in the small city we live in. He presents as more traditionally masculine than most of my clients and, as it turns out, takes declarations about the emotional tenderness of boners in stride. Mostly, he just looks relieved to have someone making definitive statements about his sex life at all. His wife of 13 years, Maria, has basically dragged him to couples therapy after two years of a drastic and unexplained decrease of sex between them and the silent, broiling resentment that's emerged as a result. To put it plainly, she's pissed—a raw state fueled by underlying emotions she reveals with little prodding: rejected, undesirable, depressed, lonely. He's apologetic, at times defensive, ashamed, and motivated by the recently realized possibility that Maria might actually leave him if sex ceases to be part of their life entirely.

It's Clark and Maria's first couples therapy session ever and, when I'm not talking about the emotional side of boners, I've been busy sketching a rough timeline of their problem story. As we do this, the three of us discover that right around the time Maria noticed that sex had "randomly dried up overnight" is also when Clark had started experiencing new-to-him erection unreliability issues. Rather than talk to Maria about his wavering erections and what might be contributing to his recent struggle to maintain them (work stress, money worries, physical exhaustion, etc.), Clark instead chose to silently make a quick-and-stoic pivot away from sex entirely. Clark had thought to himself, "Ignore the boner problem, avoid the boner problem," but in reality, he was ignoring his partner and creating a much bigger problem than a natural, understandable, and extremely common[2] change in erection patterns.

What Clark and Maria don't know (yet) is that the problem with their sex life doesn't actually revolve around Clark's hardons. It actually stems from their beliefs about hard-ons and the stories that go along with them. Clark and Maria's shared views of the role of erections in any given sexual interaction are common, highly gendered, and reliant on the myth that "sex" is entirely defined by penis-in-vagina penetration. The myth is that boners are easy, are fed by a purely biological "need" for sex, experience little influence from the outside world, and are a clear barometer for a person's desire for their partner.

As you'll recall from Chapter 1, these unfortunately misinformed stories about sex and boners weren't created by Maria or Clark. They are fueled by outside contexts, non-comprehensive sex education, gossip, shame, secrecy, and the lived experiential "proof" of Clark's up-until-now very reliable erections. Because of these stories and their shared silence about this issue, Clark and Maria have so far suffered a sexual disconnect. Clark has been busy scrambling to avoid the issue rather than challenge and work with the issue, and Maria has been (literally and figuratively) fumbling in the dark as she attempts to seduce Clark back into their sex life to no avail. When these attempts ultimately fail, Maria gets discouraged, and, just like Clark has opted to do, she turns away entirely rather than speak up about the cycle at play.

Amidst this silence, both Clark and Maria continue to operate around their shared-yet-unspoken unhelpful assumptions and understandings about erections and therefore repeatedly use Clark's boner as a barometer of their shared sexual health and connection. As Maria had said right before I made my "erections are emotional" proclamation: "Aren't men just always ready to go? What am I doing wrong? Why doesn't he want me anymore?" As Maria's statements show, Clark and Maria have clearly been silently telling themselves stories about their relationship, making unhelpful deductions from what has been left unsaid and undone in their sex life. As an important first step in their work to save their sexual connection, Maria and Clark need to bring these stories to light so they can decide where and how these internal narratives can be edited. If Clark and Maria can start speaking more openly about their sex life, they can save their shared sexual story.

Negative Narratives: When Your Problem Story Becomes Your Problem Reality

We've all got stories we tell ourselves about ourselves. Though there are many ways to tell the story, we tend to pick one way and stick to it ("I'm too anxious to try new things," "I could never start my own business," "I'm unlovable," "I'm just not like that," "If my partner isn't visibly physically aroused the minute they initiate sex, they must not be into me anymore"). When these stories are self-limiting, self-defeating, or otherwise unhelpful, therapists call them *Negative Narratives*,[3] which are, not-so-coincidentally, the narratives therapists tend to hear frequently from their clients. These types of stories hold clients back from seeing or acting on new options, dig all existing ruts a little deeper, and often need to be adjusted or retold entirely if our clients are to leave our offices feeling subjectively changed for the better (a process that usually happens through shifts in language and a process called *externalizing the problem*, which will be more thoroughly covered in Chapter 11). Typically, Negative Narratives are retold so many times to others or ourselves that we simply believe them as the truth, to be accommodated rather than challenged, scaled rather than dismantled entirely; they're good and embedded like that. These narratives can also affect how we think about ourselves as sexual people. We've all got these types of stories about sex and how we exist within our sex life. Negative Narratives can run rampant if left unchecked and, as you can imagine, negative sexual narratives are not very conducive to living your best sex life.

If Chapter 4's Pleasure Pessimism describes the collection of components that lead to a person's pleasure-sabotaging patterns (thoughts, feelings, beliefs, and actions), Negative Narratives serve as the thread that holds them all together (the motivation, plotline, and predictability of what comes next based on "who you are," "what you do," and "knowing how this will go"). Whether positive, negative, or somewhere in between, we create these narratives because that is how we make sense of the world and our place in it, and how we can fabricate an element of control over life's (or, as the case may be, our erections') unpredictable nature. Though stability and predictability can be a wonderful, positive container to many aspects of life (steady income, a reliable self-care routine, a consistent set of values you live life by), painting yourself into a corner of "what you do" in sex or "who you are" sexually is mostly just an excellent way to have some so-so sex. If we understand that relationships, desire, sex, and sexuality are inherently fluid and ever-evolving, then attempting to hold yourself stagnantly in line with your go-to Negative Narratives goes against the natural shifting of your sexual tides.

Happily, we can use cognitive behavioral therapy (CBT) to reshape our Negative Narratives from stories of Pleasure Pessimism to tales of Pleasure Optimism. In Chapter 4, we learned how CBT can help us challenge the way we think, feel, and behave in regard to our problems. CBT works against Pleasure Pessimism specifically because it views the Negative Narratives we tell about our sex lives and asks, "Really? Like, *actually* though?" It does this until we're able to see our stories through multiple lenses ("Erections don't necessarily reflect attraction," "What else could be affecting Clark's physical arousal?", "What are some other ways we can be sexual together without an erection present?") rather than the single lens we've been looking through ("Boners = sexual self-worth and level of sexual interest"). Using elements of CBT, such as evidence-gathering ("What proof do I have in my real life that my negative beliefs, fears, and stories about my sex life are true?") and exposure therapy (such as "If I ask directly for what I want during sex, will my partner actually get hurt and offended? Or might they react in a different way?"), we can challenge the validity and usefulness of our current Negative Narratives and recraft our stories away from maintaining our unsatisfying sexual status quo and toward building more flexibility, evolution, and creative problem-solving into our long-lasting, dynamic sex lives.

CBT and Your Sex Life

So far, we've been exploring the cognitive realm of how we *think* about our sex lives, our sexualities, and sex in general. It's important to talk and think about how we conceptualize sex, how we've come to know what we know, and how our outside influences have (positively or negatively) impacted those thought patterns. However, if we want to enact tangible change in our sex lives, we also need to explore how our thoughts translate into either self-limiting or self-liberating *actions*. We can't transform our Pleasure Pessimism into Pleasure Optimism without doing something differently in our actual sexual experiences. Though a cognitive shift is a very important piece of this transformative puzzle, it's not enough to simply *think* your way out of a sex rut, a pleasure-sabotaging behavior pattern, or the sinking feeling that you're just not good enough. It's important that both our thought patterns *and* our modes of behaving in sexual situations are aligned to create the conditions for truly good, authentically pleasurable sex. We can do this in a few ways:

- By allowing our new and positive thought patterns to influence our behaviors
- By experimenting with new behaviors in order to posi-

tively reinforce our new thought patterns
- By openly acknowledging the ripple effect that both positive cognition and optimistic behavior have on each other

CBT looks at the basic cycle of thought-feeling-behavior and asks, "Where can we break this pattern?" Some of these cycle components (i.e., behavior and thoughts) are easier to intentionally shift than others (i.e., core beliefs and feelings). It's much easier to change what you *do* during sex or how you *think* about yourself or your partner during sex than it is to suddenly change your complex belief systems about sex or how you feel about sex. For example, suppose someone struggles with the *thought*: "My O-face must look so stupid." It would be easier for this person to change that *thought* to something like "How I feel in my body is more important than how I look" than it would be to change their core *feeling* of self-conscious discomfort to suddenly feeling 100 percent confident in their sexual body and life. The latter would take a little more effort for most.

Because it's easier to take immediate action in the realms of your behaviors or thoughts, these are the points of entry we'll focus on when looking to take *action* to break our pleasure-pessimistic cycles. Luckily, when we shift one part of the cycle, we shift the patterned flow of all of the cycle's parts. Meaning, when we are able to change our behaviors and thoughts, our belief systems and feelings will organically follow suit without our having to exert any additional effort. This happy ripple effect will change our pleasure-pessimistic cycle as a whole and shift the Negative Narratives that go along with it.

To illustrate how these interventions might operate in real life, let's return to Jessa from Chapter 4, who is starting to resent her partner Levi for his lack of sexual intuition:

JESSA'S CYCLE OF PLEASURE PESSIMISM

Automatic Thoughts

· I wish Levi would touch my clit more but I don't know how I would tell him how to do that.

· I would be too embarrassed to ask or give him directions.

· If I did ask or give him directions, I would probably make him feel not good enough or emasculated.

· What if he thinks I haven't liked sex this entire time??

· (Because he can't read my mind) he's clearly not a very attentive lover.

· (Because he's not guessing correctly) he clearly just doesn't get me.

Negative Narrative

Levi and I don't have a very satisfying sex life and it's never going to change. He doesn't know how to pleasure me and I can't ask him to do anything differently.

Core Belief

Levi should just know how to have sex with me (but he doesn't so we're doomed).

Resulting Feelings

· Helpless
· Unsatisfied
· Unloved
· Disconnected from Levi
· Frustrated
· Almost ready to call it quits with Levi

Unhelpful Behaviors

· Doesn't ask Levi for what she wants out of sex

· Doesn't give Levi any direction or feedback

· Continues to wait for Levi to guess correctly or do something that she finds pleasurable, accidentally

· Leaves Levi in charge of their sexual dynamic

Jessa's illustration shows just one of her pleasure-pessimistic patterns of thoughts, feelings, and behaviors and the unhelpful core belief they stem from. Most of us, Jessa included, have more than one core belief about sex, spanning the spectrum of unhelpful/negative to helpful/positive. For example, alongside the idea that "Levi should just know how to have sex with me" (unhelpful/hopeless/negative), Jessa might also think, "I am deserving of a satisfying and pleasurable sex life" (helpful/motivating/positive). Problems arise when we have so many pleasure-pessimistic belief systems that we're no longer able to balance them out with positive belief systems, leading us to feel demotivated, hopeless, and trapped in one pattern of thinking.

When this happens, our pessimistic beliefs stick out in our mind, masquerading as *the truth* of our stuckness, of our short-comings, and of our partners' failures: this is the backbone of the Negative Narratives we tell ourselves, our friends, and even our therapist about our sex life. This constant retelling of our pleasure-pessimistic stories is how Negative Narratives are created and reinforced over time. Jessa has internalized a certain, well-worn story about Levi, about herself, and about their sexual partnership as a whole. To undo this toxic pattern, she must start questioning the validity of her Negative Narratives and start exploring new ways to tell her sexual story that include hope, possibility, and new avenues for solution-exploration. This is the first step for Jessa in taking pleasure-optimistic action in her sex life.

To start this questioning and retelling of her Negative Narrative, Jessa and I start by simply noticing (and writing down) the various components of her Pleasure Pessimism—the thoughts, feelings, beliefs, and actions—that she has so far taken for granted or have gone unnoticed (an insight-building process that we covered in Chapter 4). Now that she sees the pieces at play here, Jessa can choose to take new *action*: she can either modify her automatic thoughts or change her behaviors, or preferably both, as a way to transform her entire sexual story.

Change Your Pleasure-Pessimistic Thoughts

It can be intimidating to jump right into changing our sexual and relational behaviors, so when working with Jessa (and most clients), we start with questioning and modifying her limiting, pleasure-pessimistic automatic thoughts about her sex life. Thanks to Chapter 4, your unhelpful thoughts have been caught (see page 95 for a recap of your unhelpful thoughts). If you need a real-time refresher, next time you're having sex and you're feeling anxious, bored, distracted, or displeased, tune in to your thought pattern. What are you thinking about? What's running through your mind? What judgments are you casting on yourself and your partner? What assumptions are you making? When you can, jot down those thoughts! Then read over your list and look for themes. Any core beliefs, perhaps, that these thoughts are pointing to? In Jessa's case, her automatic thoughts of "I wish Levi would touch my clit more but I don't know how to tell him that," "He's not a very attentive lover," and "He just doesn't get me" have left all of the actions she could take to change the course of her sex life in Levi's hands, not hers. Her perspective has been limited by her core belief that "Levi [read: men] should just know how to have sex with me [read: with their partners]." Playing by the unspoken rules of this core belief, Jessa's automatic thoughts don't contain any new options she could take to modify her sex

Your turn! This one is for the visual learners. Using the information from the Chapter 4 exercises about the elements of your own Pleasure Pessimism, draw your own map of how your pleasure-pessimistic thoughts, feelings, behaviors, and beliefs have influenced and been influenced by an ongoing Negative Narrative you may be stuck in in your own sex life using the blank copy of Jessa's map below.

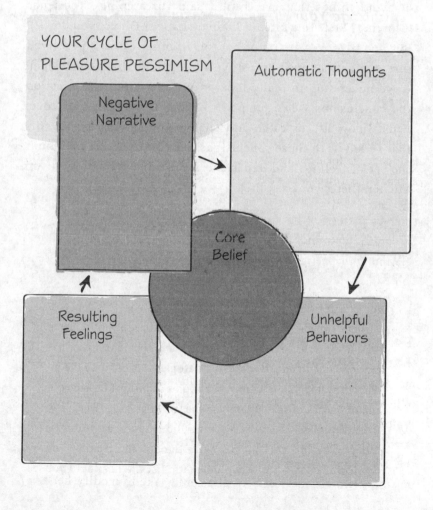

YOUR CYCLE OF
PLEASURE PESSIMISM

Negative
Narrative

Automatic Thoughts

Core
Belief

Resulting
Feelings

Unhelpful
Behaviors

life with Levi, and because Levi isn't magically guessing correctly at what Jessa wants, Jessa has been looking at Levi's sexual partnership through snot-colored glasses (that's the official opposite of rose-colored glasses, right?).

Our survival instincts rightfully encourage us to be on alert for threats so that we can either learn from a threatening experience (Ouch! I'm not touching a hot stove ever again!) or avoid things that may repeat said threatening experience (Glowing? Red? In a kitchen? Stove-shaped? Oh no, you don't!). But not all stoves are on or hot, or, in other cases, a perceived threat might not even be a stove at all (Dude, that's the fridge). If we never stop to really look at our surroundings, question the conclusions we've jumped to (That fridge is a hot stove; I just know it!), or catch and change the automatic thoughts that've led us to those conclusions, we can unnecessarily limit the set of feelings and experiences we can have in any given kitchen (here, your sex life).

A Note on Protective Pessimism

Not all automatic, pessimistic thoughts and behaviors concerning your sex life, the world, or your place in it are *bad*. Some pessimistic ways of thinking about sex and relationships or behaving within them are **adaptive strategies** designed by the intelligent system of our brains and bodies to protect us from our subjective lack of sexual safety in the world at large (which can be heavily influenced by race, gender, body type, sex, sexuality, traumatic events, etc.). As you move through this chapter, you may identify some **protective thoughts** that are helpful to you alongside of pleasure-pessimistic thoughts that are unhelpful and hindering you from pleasure, the Authentic Mood, and genuine communication.

The latter are what we will be focusing on getting out of the way. The former, if you've identified them as helpful, necessary, and protective, should be kept in place as you see fit. What I want is for you to unpack the extra, useless bricks in your sexual backpack that are weighing you down—not toss out the water, food, and first aid kit that keep you safe—or safer—on your journey. If you think that an automatic thought or behavior might indeed be protective rather than simply pleasure-pessimistic, note it here to explore in a more professional setting outside of what this book can offer.

When we slow down our well-worn threat recordings, especially when we can do so far enough away from an active kitchen (here, thinking or talking about sex outside of an actively sexual context), we are able to have the space and the time to ask ourselves the questions: Do my core beliefs and thoughts about this situation actually apply here? How do they? How don't they? If they don't, how have they been negatively impacting my sex life? What would change for the better if I were to adjust my thoughts accordingly? CBT and I help Jessa do this in her sessions.

Jessa *does* have options in her sex life with Levi, she just hasn't written them into her story yet. According to CBT, one way we can modify our automatic thoughts is by gathering evidence for and against those thoughts as we question their creation, validity, and impact. Though many have tried to shift their limiting ways of thinking about sex *during* sex, this often isn't a successful approach, understandably so. You're facing your automatic thoughts in real time and taking actions related to those thoughts; you're turned on, you're naked, you're excited, you're nervous, you're in all kinds of vulnerable emotional and physical states. If we can slow down, back up, and get some space between us and a sexual moment, we'll better be able to get a sense of what our automatic thoughts are rooted in and what core beliefs they point to, and constructively question their contribution to our most pleasure-optimistic sex life. You can do this here, right now, with this worksheet.

Challenge and Modify Your Automatic Thoughts

List any themes or core beliefs you've found in your list of automatic thoughts:

Jessa's core belief: Levi should just know how to have sex with me and know what I want.

Your Unhelpful Automatic Thoughts (see page 95 in Chapter 4 or make a new list!)

Jessa's automatic thoughts:

- *I wish Levi would touch my clit more, but I don't know how I would tell him how to do that.*
- *I would be too embarrassed to ask or give him directions.*
- *(Because he's not guessing correctly) he clearly just doesn't get me.*

Some Guiding Questions to Help Challenge Your Automatic Thoughts and Core Beliefs:

1. What facts or lived experiences support these thoughts?

2. What existing evidence contradicts it?

3. What assumptions am I making that are influencing these thoughts?

4. What would the worst possible outcome be if my thoughts came true? How would I respond, cope, or react?

5. Am I using a past experience either with this partner or past partners to overgeneralize? If so, describe that experience briefly below, noting any places that might not hold true to your current experiences.

6. What outside influences taught me to think this way about myself, about sex, or about my partner? Do I trust them? Are they reliable?

7. What are my reliable, trusted, or idolized sexual resources or examples? What would they say about my situation and thoughts? What advice would they give?

8. What advice would I give a friend in this same situation with these same thoughts?

9. What are my personal sexual values, visions, and goals? How are these thoughts supporting or sabotaging those values, visions, and goals?

Consider your responses to the questions above. Now, return to your list of automatic thoughts and modify them accordingly to reflect any positive, pleasure-optimistic notions contained in your above responses. Your glasses don't have to be perfectly rose-colored yet, but hopefully they're a few shades brighter than they were before.

Here's how Jessa's modified automatic thoughts might look:

Jessa's Modified Automatic Thoughts

Unchecked, Unhelpful Thought	New, Checked, and Modified Thought
I wish Levi would touch my clit more, but I don't know how I would tell him how to do that.	I don't know how to tell him how to do that yet, but I could feel more confident in doing this with some self-exploration of how I like to be touched and with some practice in giving him direction with other kinds of intimate or nonsexual touch.
I would be too embarrassed to ask or give him directions.	I might be embarrassed at first, but I don't think he would ridicule me or add to my embarrassment. Giving him verbal direction or feedback would likely get easier with practice, but I won't know until I start.
If I did ask or give him directions, I would probably make him feel not good enough or emasculated.	I don't know that Levi would actually feel this way. I could check in with him in the moment or after to see how it made him feel. And if he did feel not good enough or emasculated, we could talk about that together. We've successfully repaired hurt feelings and conflict before.
What if he thinks I haven't liked sex this entire time?	I don't know that Levi would actually think this way. I could ask him if he does or offer reassurance that this isn't true. I think this is something we could work through.

(Because he can't read my mind) he's clearly not a very attentive lover.	It's unfair to expect Levi to read my mind (he doesn't do so in other areas of our life, so why would he in our sex life?). If I let Levi know what I want and like and he still doesn't make an effort, then I might have reason to believe he's not attentive as a sexual partner and then I could reevaluate our relationship more critically.
(Because he's not guessing correctly) he clearly just doesn't get me.	Levi does get me in a lot of ways. If I don't give him the information he needs to get me sexually, it's likely I'll continue to feel misunderstood by him.

Your Turn! Modify Those Thoughts!

Unchecked, Unhelpful Thought	New, Checked, and Modified Thought

Unchecked, Unhelpful Thought	New, Checked, and Modified Thought

Take Action!

Small steps lead to big changes, and every shift you make in your sex life will have a ripple effect on the pleasure-pessimistic cycles at play. Below, list one small action you can take immediately in the arena of shifting your thoughts:

Next time I notice myself thinking _____, I'm going to tell myself _____ instead.

Below is an illustration of how this simple shift in automatic thought patterns might positively influence Jessa's sex life and the Negative Narratives that have been dominating her sexual story.

JESSA'S CYCLE OF PLEASURE
PESSIMISM w/ Modified
Automatic Thoughts

Automatic Thoughts

- I wish Levi would touch my clit more, but I don't know how I would tell him how to do that.

Changed to:

- I don't know how to tell him how to do that yet but I could feel more confident in doing this with some self-exploration of how I like to be touched and with some practice in giving him direction with other kinds of intimate or nonsexual touch. The only way I'll learn is to try.

Negative Narrative

Levi and I don't have a very satisfying sex life and it's never going to change **(change is possible!)**. He doesn't know how to pleasure me **(he might not know yet but can learn with my input!)** and I can't ask him to do anything differently **(I can, it just makes me a little nervous to speak up!)**.

Core Belief Shift

Levi intuitively knowing how to have sex with me isn't the marker of our sexual success. His listening and actively responding to my intel about how I like to be touched is.

Resulting Feelings

- Helpless
- Unsatisfied

Changed to:

- Nervous yet excited to have tried a new thing
- Hopeful for more positive change in the future
- More sexually satisfied
- More connected to Levi from having expressed her actual need and observing him trying to please her

Unhelpful Behaviors

- Doesn't ask Levi for what she wants out of sex
- Doesn't give Levi any direction or feedback

Changed to:

- Gives Levi a basic direction: "Could you actually add more pressure and slow down? Yes! Like that!"

Your turn! Using your small, actionable step in the arena of shifting your automatic thoughts, play around with how this small modification might have a positive ripple effect in your sex life or relationship/s.

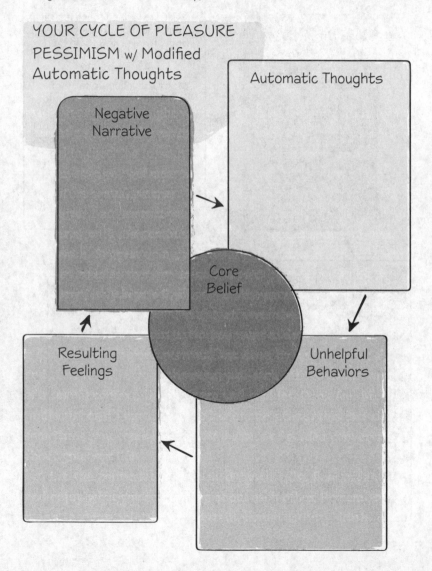

YOUR CYCLE OF PLEASURE
PESSIMISM w/ Modified
Automatic Thoughts

Negative
Narrative

Automatic Thoughts

Core
Belief

Resulting
Feelings

Unhelpful
Behaviors

Change Your Pleasure-Sabotaging Behaviors

Our actions and inactions have the power to confirm or deny our own Negative Narratives and Pleasure Pessimism. As we can see from Jessa's story, continuing to stay silent about the kind of sexual touch and experience she wants to have with Levi creates and reinforces her unhelpful thoughts and beliefs. In the case of Clark and Maria, Clark's choice to turn away from Maria rather than turn toward her in sharing his experience internally confirms for him that he doesn't get to have sexual or emotional connection without reliable erections. Maria's choice to continue to fruitlessly come on to Clark as an attempted solution rather than shifting to verbal problem-solving has only left her sexless and exasperated.

When Jessa, Maria, Clark, and the rest of us are able to change the way we think about sex during, before, and after sex, we will likely inherently shift the way we are acting in our sex lives. However, we can also shift our actions in order to shift our thoughts or, better yet, do a combination of both. Often, we haven't yet spontaneously changed our current sexual behavior patterns because the risk of such a shift feels greater than the possible reward. Jessa fears she'll be embarrassed or injure Levi's sexual ego or sense of (socially defined) masculinity. Clark fears feelings of inadequacy, judgment, and shame if he confesses to Maria that his erections haven't been as reliable as in the past. Maria fears rejection due to what she assumes is Clark's loss of sexual interest in her so her strategy is to double-down on her sexual efforts. As I like to ask my clients when they come in with a problem story featuring their own unhelpful, repeated actions:

"So, is [insert unhelpful yet relentlessly repeated action here] working for you so far?"

"Jessa, is staying silent about what you want from sex
working for you so far?"

"Maria, is continuing to wordlessly initiate sex with Clark
working so far?"

"Clark, is ignoring your erection loss and the feelings this
brings up working so far?"

"Hey, you reading this book, is _____ working so far?"

Chances are that, no, it is not. It's admittedly quite hard to
take new actions that you can't yet see as possibilities, an issue
almost all of us have in at least some area of our lives because
we are just so close to our own issues that we can't zoom out
far enough to see any alternatives (this is usually where therapists or sometimes even just a blunt friend can come in handy).
It's easier to see new action possibilities when we are able to
label our current behavior patterns as the unhelpful and unchallenged habits they have become, and are able to track and
shift the ripple effect they have as just one cog in the well-oiled
thought-feeling-behavior machine. When we do this, we can ask
ourselves, "Huh, I wonder why I keep doing this super unhelpful and pleasure-sabotaging thing in my sex life when it's obviously not working?" (Spoiler alert: usually it's fear of judgment,
rejection, or abandonment). Then we can get to the business of
acting brave.

As Ralph Waldo Emerson famously said, "A hero is no braver
than an ordinary [person], but [they are] brave five minutes
longer."[4,5] When thinking about taking new action to shift old
behaviors in your sex life, consider the actions you could take
in five minutes or less ("Telling my girlfriend I'm into kink,"
"Doing a quick Google about that sex thing I think I'm into,"
"Trying on the lingerie I worried was 'too slutty'") or break

your new action into five-minute pieces ("Telling my girlfriend I'm into kink," then "Managing my anxiety about her reaction," then "Initiating a follow-up talk about our boundaries, resources, and what we might be willing to try together"). Most of us will find that acting brave for just five minutes rarely leads to the disaster our anxious minds have convinced us will surely come (officially called *catastrophizing* in CBT) and rather is more likely to lead us to new evidence that advocating for our pleasure will better guide us to where, how, and with whom we can safely and consensually explore that pleasure. In the activity "The Business of Acting Brave," you can discover five minutes of bravery in your sex life.

The Business of Acting Brave

What's my repeated, unhelpful behavior that I just keep frickin' doing?

Jessa's example: Staying quiet about what I actually want out of sex, during sex.

What's the fear that I'm avoiding by continuing this behavior?

Jessa's example: Embarrassment, hurting Levi's feelings, temporary tension in our sex life.

Is this fear real, backed up by present-day experience, protecting me from real threat or harm? (If you answer *yes* to this question, then this behavior may be in place for a very good reason and should be addressed with a professional or as a symptom of abuse or trauma, not here in this book with a worksheet.)

Jessa's example: No, I'm confident that talking about our sex life with Levi would be a baseline safe thing to do.

Is this fear based on a past experience? Do you think it may repeat in your present-day relationship? What do you think is most likely to happen in your present-day relationship?

Jessa's example: Yes, my ex did respond to my sexual feedback with hurt feelings, shutting down, and tension, but I'm not sure Levi would do the same thing. I am worried that I will feel embarrassed or not know how to have this conversation.

If I were to act with five minutes of bravery, what are three new and different behaviors I could try, immediately, in five minutes or less?

Jessa's example: I could suggest we go sex toy shopping! I could ask him if we could make a drink-coffee-and-discuss-our-sex-life date soon! I could give him some simple requests during sex that seem easier (like "slower," "to the left," "like that," etc.).

What are the possible positive ramifications of this shiny new behavior? What would be the worst possible outcome? What do I think is actually the most likely outcome?

Jessa's responses:

Positives: More communication between us. Less mind-reading for Levi. Greater chances of a satisfying sex life and relationship overall.

Worst possible: I take a risk and act in a new, empowered way. Levi reacts by shutting down or being hurt, or maybe doesn't adjust his behavior at all. I end up mortified, telling myself "I told you so."

Most likely: I feel awkward and nervous saying something. Levi responds to the best of his ability. We see how it goes, maybe we process it a little afterward and we get better at this new system over time with practice.

Positives:

Worst possible:

Most likely:

If my worst possible outcome did indeed happen, what would I do and how would I cope?

Jessa's example: Ride out the awkwardness, confide in a trusted friend about it, find a way to talk about sex that works for us both.

Take Action!

When we continue to take the same unhelpful actions or respond in the same way to our partners' actions in our sex lives, it's likely that we'll continue to get the same unwanted results. Below, list one small action you can take immediately in the arena of shifting your pleasure-sabotaging behaviors in your sex life:

Next time I notice myself doing _____, I'm going to do _____ instead.

Below is an illustration of how trying one of her new, brave behaviors in her sex life might shift the entire pleasure-pessimistic thought-feeling-behavior cycle for Jessa.

JESSA'S CYCLE OF PLEASURE PESSIMISM
w/ Modified Behaviors

Automatic Thoughts

- I wish Levi would touch my clit more, but I don't know how I would tell him how to do that.
- (Because he can't read my mind) he's clearly not a very attentive lover.
- (Because he's not guessing correctly) he clearly just doesn't get me.

Changed to:

- We're both on this sexual journey of learning new things about our sexual pleasure together.
- It's not that he doesn't care or isn't a good lover, he just hasn't had the info (and I haven't had all of the info either!).
- I don't have to be the only one giving Levi new sexual information; we can also seek out that info from other sources and learn together.

Negative Narrative Shift

Levi and I don't have a very satisfying sex life **(our current sex life iteration no longer works and we need an update!)** and it's never going to change **(change is possible!)**. He doesn't know how to pleasure me and I can't ask him to do anything differently. **(With new info, he may change on his own!)**

Core Belief Shift

Knowledge about sexual pleasure and what makes for good sex is a constantly evolving process, not an inherently "known," one-time download.

Resulting Feelings

- Helpless
- Disconnected from Levi

Changed to:

- Nervous yet excited to have tried a new thing
- Connected to Levi with a fun, shared experience
- On a collaborative playing field as we both learn new info about sexual pleasure at the toy shop

Unhelpful Behaviors

- Continues to wait for Levi to guess correctly or do something that she finds pleasurable, accidentally
- Leaves Levi in charge of their sexual dynamic

Changed to:

- "Hey Levi, I think it would be super fun to go to a sex toy shop and learn about some new sexy things we can do!"

Your turn! Using your small, actionable step in the arena of shifting your unhelpful behaviors, play around with how this modification might have a positive ripple effect in your sex life or relationship(s) with the blank map below.

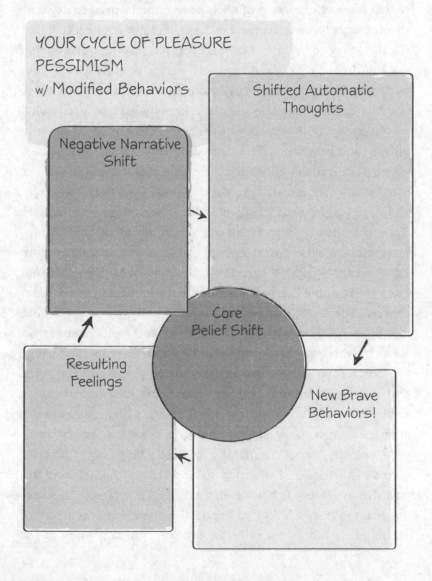

YOUR CYCLE OF PLEASURE PESSIMISM
w/ Modified Behaviors

Shifted Automatic Thoughts

Negative Narrative Shift

Core Belief Shift

Resulting Feelings

New Brave Behaviors!

Sometimes once we are able to identify why we continue to behave in a certain way and get a fuller picture of the ripple effects of our go-to actions in our sex lives, we are struck by a bolt of motivation that then shifts that behavior easily in our next sexual interactions. Most of us, however, might need to do some smaller steps toward change. For Jessa, it might not be likely that she'll just say to herself, "Oh yes, I see that staying quiet during sex isn't helping me," and then will decide to start giving Levi feedback, direction, and suggestions like an old pro. For Clark and Maria, they might decide, "You know what, the patriarchal reinforcement of the erection as the centerpiece of sex *is* actually bullshit and now we will act in accordance with our own values, which place our shared, shifting pleasure at the center of our sex life instead!" Or, more likely, these clients, you, your partner(s), and even I might need a little practice at behaving with Pleasure Optimism before we truly hit our stride. By using the CBT intervention called *exposure therapy* (don't worry, it sounds more sinister than it is), we can break our new behavior goals into more manageable pieces, which not only helps us collect valuable real-life proof that we can act differently with success but also bolsters our motivation and sense of accomplishment as we check off these new tasks and build greater sexual self-esteem.

When something gives a client fear or anxiety to the point that they avoid it entirely, they do not have any opportunities to disprove their negative feelings. Exposure therapy gradually exposes a client to something that gives them fear and/or anxiety. Typically, exposure therapy is used to help clients practice pieces of their feared situation to help reduce the negative impact this avoidance is having on their life. For example, if someone wanted or needed more financial income but was afraid of asking their boss for a raise, in exposure therapy they might start with smaller self-advocating actions that would help them practice for the big ask, like directly asking for correct change if a shop teller were to make a mistake or asking their procrastinating co-worker to promptly complete a task for a shared project. Gradually, this person would practice the self-advocating and direct-communication components of the task "ask my boss for a raise" in lower-stakes scenarios until they had enough lived experience and self-confidence that they could reasonably face the (hopefully now lowered) anxiety about asking their boss for a raise.

The vast majority of my clients describe anxiety and fear around asking for what they want, wanting what they want, and taking consensual action toward what they want in their sex lives. When left unchecked, these common anxieties and fears can become looming barricades between individuals and their sexual satisfaction. Exposure therapy can be utilized to identify and face these fears and anxieties that hold so many back from taking action. By identifying the underlying triggers embedded in your problem-saturated sexual interaction or thought pattern and then creating a list of smaller, relevant actions to practice (either in or outside of your actual sex life), you can chip away at the barriers between you and your desired sex life goal until your goal seems manageably tackled with just five minutes of bravery.

Gradual Exposure Therapy for Your Sex Life

It's important to note that exposure therapy, in any area of your life but especially in your sex life, is done with your own (and, when relevant, your partner's) willing consent. Meaning, exposure therapy is not the following approach: "I'm afraid of oranges so I'm going to jump into a ball pit of oranges, have a complete meltdown, and fear-attack the entire time in the name of 'therapy.'" That's just horrible and traumatizing. Instead, exposure therapy needs to be *gradual* exposure to elements of the thing you want to de-crease your fear of—elements that you choose for yourself (through collaboration with a therapist or a sexual partner who can help you generate ideas) and at a pace that you choose for yourself. Here's how you might do this in your sex life, using Maria and Clark's couples therapy goals as an example:

1. **Identify your new behavior goal.**

Clark's example: Have a fulfilling, anxiety-free sexual encounter with Maria, whether or not my erection is present or reliable.

2. What is the theme of this goal?

Clark's example: Be present and proactive in our sex life, even when my body isn't doing exactly what I want it to do. Accept my body as it is and for what it can or can't do.

3. Make a list of 5–10 things you could try in or outside of your sex life that would help you work toward this new behavior goal. (See table on page 159.)

Clark's list:

1. *Co-create a plan with Maria to have sex without erections being part of it at all.*

2. *Talk to two trusted, nonjudgmental friends about their experiences with erection un/reliability, masculinity, and social stigma to seek validation and support.*

3. *Directly ask Maria for different sexual touch when my erection falters.*

4. *Tell Maria directly and verbally if I'm just not in the sexual mood and practice managing my own reactions to her possible disappointment.*

5. *Shop for sex toys we could use together if Maria wants the type of penetration my erection provides when it's not around to provide it.*

1.

2.

3.

4.

5.

6.

7.

8.

9.

10.

4. Give each item a rating on a scale of 1–10 about how much anxiety you think taking this action might cause you (1 = none and 10 = SO MUCH).

5. Make a timing plan. You can either take these new actions as they come up organically, or you can plot them out in your calendar—for example, taking one new action once a week.

6. As you take each new action, check them off your list and then re-rate them on the same scale of 1–10 but this time, your rating will be how much anxiety taking the new action *actually* caused you in real life.

My Exposure Therapy Log			
New Behavior Step	**Anxiety Prediction Rating 1–10**	**Anxiety Rating, Real Life 1–10**	**Notes:**
Clark's example: Directly ask Maria for different sexual touch when my erection falters.	8	5	Maria was way more engaged with this than I thought she would be! I do want to set aside some time to make a list of different types of touch I might want in the future so I more readily know what to ask for next time.

New Behavior Step	Anxiety Prediction Rating 1–10	Anxiety Rating, Real Life 1–10	Notes:

Clark and Maria fired me eight weeks after their first session. No, it's not because I told Clark that he just needs to let his boner express its pent-up emotions—they just didn't need my help anymore. One of the funny things about being a couples therapist is that being fired (in this way, at least) is ultimately the goal, so I'm always pleased to hear a client tell me, "I think we might be done here." Through their hard work in weekly couples therapy sessions and their devotion to out-of-session homework and experiments, Clark and Maria retold the Negative Narratives they had been subconsciously subscribing to about their sex life. They challenged the modern mythology we're told about what counts as sex and the exaggerated role a super-hard, reliable dick plays in those stories. They examined how these stories have been handed down to them from media, sex ed, and peers, and how they themselves had been accidentally bolstering these untrue and unhelpful tales with their own fears of rejection, fears of undesirability, shame, and silence.

By modifying both their individual thoughts and behaviors as well as the ways they had been supporting these Negative Narratives through their mutual relationship dynamic, Maria and Clark were able to simply make space for a new telling of the same problem, making it not so much of a problem after all. With a list of exciting sex acts they can do boner-free, new understandings of what *actually* signals their sexual attraction to each other, a standing policy to openly talk about the circumstances surrounding any future sexual issues, and the freeing ability to create a sex life that actually works for the two of them (and not what they've been told should work for everyone), Clark and Maria attended their last session with reports of decreased distress, increased emotional closeness, and—oh hey, would you look at that—more frequent erections for Clark, which I would call far from coincidental.

Jessa's Sexual Needs, Clark's Boners, and You
Applying CBT IRL

Any of these interventions can be done by individuals who are partnered, dating, or single, or by couples, partners, or fuck buddies. These are skills that can be worked on solo while you're not sexually active, they can be practiced via masturbation, or they can be worked on together as partners. They can be worked on by one individual in a partnership and, even if your partner does nothing to change their role in the cycle at all, change will happen in your shared sex life. The truth is that *you* can take independent action over how you think and behave (and, therefore, according to CBT theory, how you feel and what you believe) in your sex life. Just as Jessa did in her individual therapy sessions, doing this work will change the pattern that has been happening in your sex life because *you* have changed your contribution to it. When Jessa started asking more directly for what she wanted during sex with Levi, he listened. When he didn't get it quite right the first or even the second time, Jessa was able to offer him continued feedback far more easily than she thought she would. Levi directly benefited from Jessa's work and even began doing some of his own. When it was no longer an option for them to just pretend their sex life was always satisfying, Levi felt invited to consider the things *he* wanted to ask for and, with the example set by Jessa of how to ask and give feedback without being overly critical (more on this in Chapter 8), Levi felt better equipped to share more about his own complex desires with Jessa as well.

Of course, these happy endings don't always happen when we begin to examine and shift our unhelpful thoughts and habits. Sometimes you get up the gall to ask for something, give direction, or encourage your partner to correct course, and they act like a total asshole. Or, sometimes popping the bubble of "Whatever you intuitively do during sex is just fine, dear" does indeed poison the relationship beyond recovery. Sure, this can be challenging, frustrating or sometimes heartbreaking, but the pursuit of our authentic sexuality can sometimes lead us to a fork in the pleasure path where you and your partner(s) decide to go your separate ways. Ultimately, I think this is okay. I'm of the professional opinion that a split made by informed decisions and thorough self-investigation can be considered a therapeutic success when done well, but we'll get deeper into these ideas of navigating desire differences and boundary-clashes later in Chapters 9, 10, and 11.

In the end, CBT is designed to support people in creating change, both intentional and, at times, unforeseen. CBT's interventions, like noticing and challenging our automatic thoughts, gathering experiential evidence, or engaging in gradual exposure therapy, work to adjust key pieces of our pleasure-pessimistic cycle with the understanding that an adjustment to one piece will organically adjust the whole. As I like to remind my clients, this is not a magical process that will happen overnight. Core beliefs and Negative Narratives are born out of often subconscious repetition of Pleasure Pessimism and lived experiences that have "proven true" our sexual fears, hang-ups, and anxieties. This doesn't mean that these thoughts, feelings, behaviors, beliefs, and stories are impossible to change, but it does mean that a similar experience of *repeated* positive experiences will be needed to change course toward Pleasure Optimism. Like all things in our authentically pleasurable and genuine sex lives, I recommend you take the journey of reshaping your Negative Narratives toward Pleasure Optimism languidly, enjoying the unpredictable, exciting novelty that harnessing the power of your pleasure-centering thoughts and behaviors can bring to your sexual beliefs, feelings, and relationships.

The difficult internal work contained in Part 2 is, happily, not where your journey to sexual authenticity climaxes. In fact, for many people, the climaxes are just getting started. Because you've done the work of lowering the barriers listed in Part 2 (if not moving them aside entirely)—the demands of the Classic Mood, the grip of Pleasure Pessimism, and the fables contained in our old Negative Narratives—you've cleared the mental and emotional space needed to create the hot, juicy, connected, satisfying, exploratory sex life you actually want. With the skill-building elements of Part 3—desire discovery, confident sexual communication, and effective sex and relationship troubleshooting—the theory of your most pleasurable sex life can now be put into practice.

The Brain-Boner Connection
And What to Do When Your Body (Regardless of Your Type of Anatomy!) Isn't Showing Up to Sex How You'd Like It To

Of course, erections (or vaginal lubrication, for that matter) ar en't *always* linked to our emotional state. Sometimes, physical sexual issues are exactly that: physical. If you're someone who is managing erectile dysfunction, whether it's been ongoing or has come on suddenly, it's important that you evaluate *both* the possible emotional *and* physical contributors. Physically, erectile dysfunction can be a sign of heart disease, blood pressure issues, diabetes, and other serious medical conditions,[6] so it's always important to get checked by a doctor first (and for the therapists out there, it's important we recommend that our clients take this step before we dive into the psychological aspects).

Medication is often prescribed as a quick fix to erection dissatisfaction *instead of* encouraging people to explore emotional influences at play. Though erection-inducing medications are a tempting option that many people decide to take, it can be just as important to look at the emotional, mental, and relational contributors to the issue. Whether you decide to use medication or not, repairing some of the toxic thought-feeling-behavior patterns that may be sustaining your erectile dysfunction can be a helpful part of making your overall sexual relationships better, more pleasurable, and more fulfilling; remember, the presence or absence of an erection (or the presence or absence of vaginal wetness, for that matter) doesn't flawlessly correlate[7] to pleasure, consent, attraction to your partner, or emotional and sexual health. Doing a full assessment of your health, happiness, and physical, medical, mental, emotional, and relational patterns is a great holistic approach to erectile issues—and all arousal issues, no matter your body type or sexual anatomy.

If you do decide to look at the emotional factors to your erectile dysfunction, here are some places to investigate for yourself or with your partner(s):

- Evaluate your stress and sleep. Overworking, obsessing over the current news cycle, lack of rest, unhealthy sleep, or deficiencies in healthy exercise habits strain your entire body, your sexual body included. What needs to shift outside of your sex life to support your body during sex?

- De-stress before sex. Do you engage in enough self-care or daily body movement or exercise? Are you spending enough time connecting to your partner(s) emotionally or relationally before you have sex? Are you stuck scrolling screens or engaging in other distractions during the times you usually have sex? Cut those habits back and see if this shifts how you show up to sex.

- Smooth out residual relational strife. Broken trust, unresolved conflicts, stewing resentments, and ongoing unhealthy relationship dynamics, even if not directly on your mind, can show up in your bed. If you notice that this physical pattern seems to be connected to intrusive thoughts about a problem rooted in the relationship itself, it may be time to have some bigger conversations, possibly with a couples therapist.

■ Interrupt performance anxiety. Have a couple of run-ins with a faltering erection scared you into a self-fulfilling pattern of erectile dysfunction? If you notice an erection isn't coming up when you want it to, take the pressure off immediately. Don't dive right into oral sex, hand jobs, or an in-depth discussion of "how to get it back." Instead, switch gears to a different sex activity, snuggle naked and talk about something else, or pause sex entirely. Many find that taking the pressure off can be a quicker fix than they think it'll be.

■ Diversify your definitions of sex. Collaborate with your partner(s) to brainstorm a list of all the great, sexy things you can do together that have nothing to do with erections. This way, you'll have some great go-to ideas of ways to play if your boner goes away. And, in the meantime, it may come back around while you're busy enjoying other things.

10 Hot Ways to Have Sex without Boners

1. With your mouth
2. With your fingers
3. With your whole frickin' hand
4. With dildos (hand-held or strapped on, made of silicone, glass, and stainless steel, oh my!)
5. With vibrator
6. With buttplugs or anal beads
7. With rope, cuffs, gags, blindfolds, hoods, and other BDSM-inspired sensation play
8. With one person masturbating while the other person watches, caresses, dirty talks, and so on

9. With dry-humping, juicy wet-humping, or otherwise sensually rubbing your bods together

10. With erotica or porn—watching it together, reading it together, or otherwise getting in that sapiosexual headspace together

Your turn! All bodies have the potential to not act the way we wish they would during sex. A simple yet powerful way to intervene when this happens is to, rather than shutting down sex and turning away from your partner entirely, make a backup plan of ways to stay connected in the sexy zone together. This helps partners avoid creating an unhelpful cycle of sexual shame and rejection in their relationship and instead offers creative ways to keep the sexual energy alive rather than bailing the second things don't go to plan.

Below, list some fun ways you and your partner might want to be sexual, intimate, or sensual together if/when your bodies aren't showing up to sex exactly the way you would like them to.

1.

2.

3.

4.

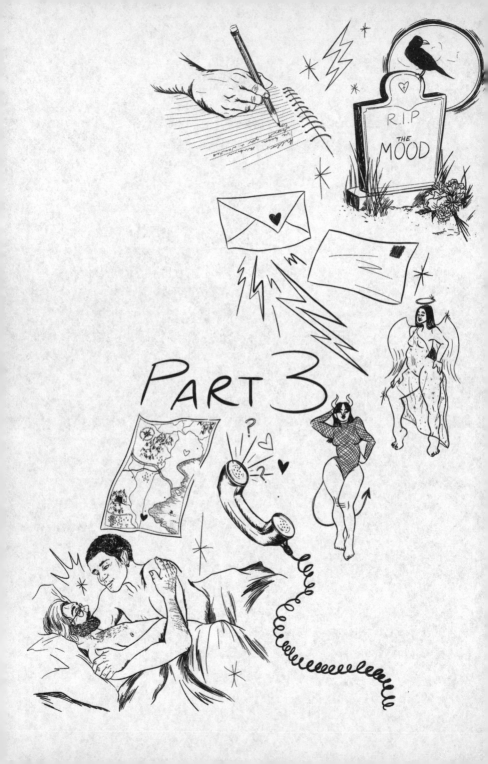

Part 3 is all about the practical application of the skills needed to create your best sex life, like how to figure out what you want out of sex, how to ask for what you want, and how to set boundaries with confidence. Part 3 is devoted to your pleasure—what it's made of, how to create space for it, how to talk about it, and how to have fun exploring it with yourself and your sexual partners.

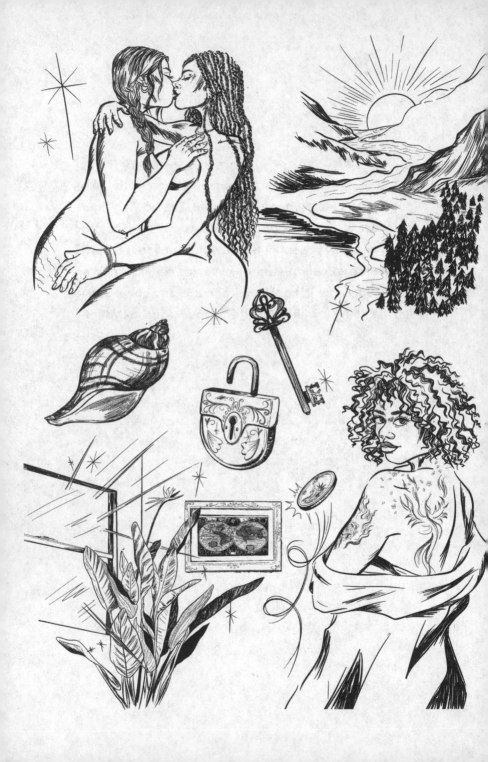

CHAPTER 6

How to Discover What You Want

*Relationships are just two people constantly asking each
other where they want to go eat, until one of them dies.*
—@robfee on Twitter, April 13, 2015

If I ask, "What do you want to eat for dinner?" some people might
have an immediate answer or craving, but many people would
likely either draw a blank, volley the question back and ask me
what *I* want for dinner, or default to a trusty go-to (mine is tacos,
always tacos). If I instead hand you two menus from my favorite
restaurants and say, "Which dishes would you like to order for
dinner? We'll go to the restaurant that sounds tastiest to you!"
you'll be greeted with an array of options that you probably
wouldn't have thought of yourself or maybe something will catch
your eye that you didn't even know was possible. Once we've actually ordered our meals at the restaurant, you might try a bite of
what I ordered and find out you like something new, something
that might even become your new favorite. Or maybe you'll try
something I love, not like it, and now know that my all-time favorite dessert (deep-fried chocolate "egg rolls," by the way) is simply not your thing (I'll never understand it, but I will, of course,
accept it).

Whether talking sex or food, it's much easier to make choices
and spark cravings when we've got a menu to choose from. How

else might you know all the ways you could have a deeply plea-surable sexual experience without knowing what is available to you in the wide, fantastic, multi-layered world of sex? The cur-rent confines of sex education and popular media certainly aren't going to present all of the options to you. And being left to think of them all by yourself is unnecessarily limiting, not to mention it's as much work as reinventing the wheel. Furthermore, if you or your partner(s) are stuck in a sex rut, having a list of options and possibilities to consider can help rekindle desire and interest in sex because most people find it challenging to organically lust after the same old sex routine.[1]

Though many of us will learn new things about our sexual selves in a sexual moment, most of us won't just stumble into this place of self-discovery without first familiarizing ourselves with the foundational basics of what we're definitely interested in, not interested in, or on the fence about. Simply put, if you want to have hot and satisfying sex, you've got to know what you want, which is easier to do with a menu! Introducing: your fully cus-tomizable menu of sexual desires, limits, and curiosities, com-monly known as the Yes/No/Maybe List.

A Yes/No/Maybe List (Y/N/M List) is exactly what you think it is: a list of sexual acts that you can mark down as "Yes—I'm into that!", "No—This is not for me!", or "Maybe—I'd be willing to try this one out or would like to know more!" A few modern versions of the Y/N/M List (including the one in this chapter) also provide additional questions that pertain to sex, such as questions about your identity, language preferences, triggers, fantasies, and sexual health. The Yes/No/Maybe List[2] isn't a new concept and is just one of many ways to explore and make new discoveries about what you want out of sex. Check out the resource guide in the back of this book for more ideas, including watching porn that depicts a variety of sex acts and dynamics, researching and exploring something you saw in a movie once, trying things your partner is into that you've yet to investigate for yourself, reading erotica, or taking a trip to your local sex toy shop to see what catches your eye.

The Y/N/M List certainly isn't the only option, but it's a piece of homework I frequently recommend to my clients and column write-ins as a helpful jumping-off point to several common sex-life conundrums: "I know asking for what I want directly is a good idea, but I don't even know what I want!", "We're stuck in a sex rut and don't really know what do to outside of the usual; got any ideas?", "I've got a new sexual partner and I don't know how to start the conversation about what their sexual boundaries are," "We want to have a threesome but don't know what our shared sexual interests are," "I feel cut off from my own sexuality and wish I knew my sexual self better." The Y/N/M List is basically my "Take two Advil and call me in the morning" remedy to many big-picture sex-life snafus. And because it's so important to know what you want, I've devoted this entire chapter to this fully customizable and original version of the Y/N/M list that I've made just for you.

There are a few ways that I recommend you use this list. First, I recommend you use it outside of a sexual context entirely. This means at your dinner table, in a cafe with your favorite espresso drink, snuggled up in your bed, or otherwise clothed, level-headed, and present. For most of us, when we are in the heat of the moment, with a lover's body all intermingling with our body, we're not in the most mentally clear space to make thoughtful decisions about our desires and boundaries. A pen-and-paper list in a nonsexual context can help us conjure the mental skills we need to focus, think things through, and create the groundwork for future in-the-moment sexual choices to be genuine, informed, and consensual.

Second, I recommend you take your first pass at this list alone rather than with a sexual partner (though, I once did a Y/N/M List with a platonic friend and that was super fun!). A solo journey through this list can make sure that you're answering based on yourself and your own wants and needs rather than what you think your partner might want to see or hear from you. If you're currently not sexually partnered, doing this list can be immensely helpful in checking in with your personal desires and boundaries and can help you get clear about what you might want to look for in a future sexual partner.

Third, I advise that you assign this list to yourself and your partner(s) (with their enthusiastic willingness, of course!) as shared homework. Suggest doing this list together as a date night, bring it up in couples therapy as an idea for between-sessions home-work, or simply blame this book for the excellent idea ("I've been reading this book about creating an awesome sex life and there's this sexual desires list in it. Do you want to do it with me?"). Pick a deadline to get your personal list done by and then set a date and time to share your answers with each other—again, outside of a sexual context, like over tea and cookies. Don't feel pressure to discuss or fill out the entire list in one sitting; this can also be something you come back to for a series of guided conversations about your sex life.

Let the conversations sparked by this list flow organically and enjoy what you're learning about each other. Remember that being incompatible about a certain sexual activity, kink, or interest isn't an automatic deal-breaker and that, just like with food, we shouldn't expect ourselves and our partners to have exactly the same likes and dislikes. It's okay to have different desires. Rather than shame or blame yourself or your partner(s) (a disconnecting experience), use this opportunity to observe where the limits lie, and where overlap occurs, and to learn new things about yourself and your partner(s) (a connecting experience). We'll get more into the nitty gritty of navigating big desire discrepancies in Chapter 11.

I also suggest you return to and update this list. Everyone's sexual desires and boundaries will evolve and shift over time because we are human beings and our bodies, relationship dynamics, circumstances, health, interests, and self-knowledge will change. If we want to have a sex life that remains satisfying for our entire lives, it's important that we tune into that evolution so that we can adapt to it. Returning to a Y/N/M List after a break-up, during a relationship transition, with a new partner (many of our boundaries will vary from partner to partner!), while recovering from infidelity, after adding a baby to the family, or even as a regular check-in with yourself can be a great way to stay up-to-date on where you stand in your own sexuality. I have even surprised myself when doing a Y/N/M List.

Finally, don't just skip this part and bank on your pleasure being a happy accident or coincidence. When it comes to your sex life, do your homework, know your options, resist limiting yourself by what you think you already know, and bring active intention to the table when creating your authentic sex life. When you do, you'll be more confident in knowing and asking for what you want, find greater ease in setting boundaries, choose partners who are truly sexually compatible with you, and, because you'll have a stronger understanding of what's sexually important to you, you'll be more resilient to rejection and sexual setbacks. Let's get to listing.

The Yes/No/Maybe List: Spark and Focus Conversations about Sex, Boundaries, and Relationships

If there's anything I want you to take away from this book, it's that your sex life can and should be customized to you and your partners and given plenty of free space to evolve. Meaning, though the Virgo rising in me loves a good checklist, nobody's sexuality can or should be reduced to the confines of neatly organized checkboxes.

This list is therefore intended to be a catalyst for sexual self-knowledge rather than a perfectly exhaustive document. Its true goal is to get you and your partner(s) thinking deeply and talking creatively about your sexual interests, boundaries, and evolutions.

This is a list to spark a conversation. If it does that, then great! If you find it too constricting, then feel free to skip over parts, modify it, write outside the margins, or add in your own options. This list, like your sexual pleasure, is *yours* after all! Whatever you do, even if you scrap this list entirely and find your own way to engage in this work, don't skip thinking about your desires and boundaries in an intentional and thoughtful way. Knowing your sexual self is an important bedrock to your authentic pleasure and your sexual communication and will go a long way in fostering both.

Language!

Language is an important part of our sex lives. It helps us communicate our desires, define ourselves, establish trust and safety, and explore our sexualities in new and complex ways. On this list, I've included certain terms for anatomy and sexual activities and I've also included blanks for self-defined anatomy vocabulary and even bigger blanks where your unique experience and imagination can fly. Feel free to skip things that simply don't apply.

Resources!

Some of these activities are higher risk than others, such as those that fall into the kinky sex categories like rope bondage and impact play. Please be sure to check out the resource guide in the back of this book for trustworthy places to gather information about this kind of sexual play. I suggest exploring higher-risk activities within a trusting and openly communicative sexual partnership.

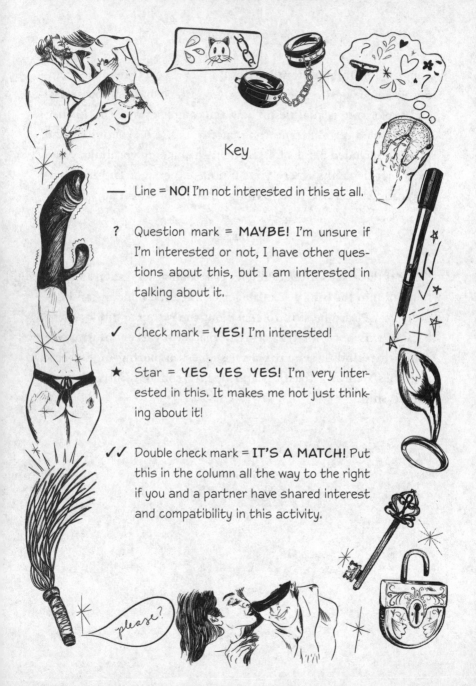

Key

— Line = **NO!** I'm not interested in this at all.

? Question mark = **MAYBE!** I'm unsure if I'm interested or not, I have other questions about this, but I am interested in talking about it.

✓ Check mark = **YES!** I'm interested!

★ Star = **YES YES YES!** I'm very interested in this. It makes me hot just thinking about it!

✓✓ Double check mark = **IT'S A MATCH!** Put this in the column all the way to the right if you and a partner have shared interest and compatibility in this activity.

please?

Yes/No/Maybe List

Activity	Solo	Giving/partnered	Receiving/partnered	Giving + receiving/partnered	Questions, concerns, notes	✓✓
					If sharing and comparing your lists with a partner, put a double check mark here if you've got compatible interest in this activity.	
Holding hands						
Massage						
Erotic massage						
Kissing						
Hot and heavy make-out session						
Touching breasts/chest						
External genital stimulation over clothes						

Activity	Solo	Giving/partnered	Receiving/partnered	Giving + receiving/partnered	Questions, concerns, notes	✓✓
External genital stimulation under clothes	·					
Dry humping						
Tribadism (rubbing naked genitals together—hint: try adding lube!)						
Using a vibrator						
Using a strap-on dildo						
Using a hand-held dildo/ vibrator for penetration						
Using a masturbation sleeve						

Activity	Solo	Giving/partnered	Receiving/partnered	Giving + receiving/partnered	Questions, concerns, notes	✓✓
Using an anal plug						
Using a dildo or vibrator anally						
Using a dildo or vibrator on/in ___						
Vulva stimulation with hands (external)						
Vaginal fingering (internal)						
Anal stimulation with hands (external)						

Activity	Solo	Giving/partnered	Receiving/partnered	Giving + receiving/partnered	Questions, concerns, notes	✓✓
Anal fingering (internal)						
Stimulation with hands on penis						
Stimulation with hands on testes/balls						
Stimulation with hands on _____ _____						
Stimulation with mouth/ tongue on/in anus						
Stimulation with mouth/ tongue on/ in vulva and vagina						

Activity	Solo	Giving/partnered	Receiving/partnered	Giving + receiving/partnered	Questions, concerns, notes	✓✓
Stimulation with mouth/ tongue on penis						
Stimulation with mouth/ tongue on testes/balls						
Stimulation with mouth/ tongue on _____ _____						
69ing (mutual, simultaneous oral sex)						
Clitoral stimulation with toys						
Clitoral stimulation with hands						

Activity	Solo	Giving/partnered	Receiving/partnered	Giving + receiving/partnered	Questions, concerns, notes	✓✓
Vaginal penetration with a strap-on dildo or penis						
Anal penetration with a strap-on dildo or penis						
Other penetrative sex (get specific in the notes section about where and with what)						
Vaginal fisting						
Anal fisting						

Activity	Solo	Giving/partnered	Receiving/partnered	Giving + receiving/partnered	Questions, concerns, notes	✓✓
_____ fisting						
Ejaculation on someone's body (get specific as to where in the notes)						
Ejaculation inside someone's body (get specific as to where in the notes)						
Mutual masturbation with a partner						
Masturbation alone						

Activity	Solo	Giving/partnered	Receiving/partnered	Giving + receiving/partnered	Questions, concerns, notes	✓✓
Dirty talk						
Sexting (specify text, photos, videos, voice messages)						
Phone sex (verbal, no video)						
Video chat sex (i.e., Skype or FaceTime)						
Reading erotica alone						
Reading erotica with a partner						
Watching porn alone						

Activity	Solo	Giving/partnered	Receiving/partnered	Giving + receiving/partnered	Questions, concerns, notes	✓✓
Watching porn with a partner						
Watching porn with a partner while having sex/being sexual						
Threesomes or group sex (get specific in the notes)						
Dressing up for sex (specify in the notes)						
Bondage with rope						

Activity	Solo	Giving/partnered	Receiving/partnered	Giving + receiving/partnered	Questions, concerns, notes	✓✓
Bondage with other restraints						
Blindfolding						
Covering mouth with hands						
Ball gags (specify wearing or wanting partner to wear)						
Leaving marks (specify where and how)						
Slapping (specify where)						

Activity	Solo	Giving/partnered	Receiving/partnered	Giving + receiving/partnered	Questions, concerns, notes	✓✓
Spanking						
Flogging						
Choking (This is a HIGH-RISK activity and should only be done after proper education within a trusted sexual partnership)						
Biting						
Spitting/ drooling						
Scratching						
Rough body play						

Activity	Solo	Giving/partnered	Receiving/partnered	Giving + receiving/partnered	Questions, concerns, notes	✓✓
Voyeurism (watching others be sexual/have sex, specify)						
Exhibitionism (being watched being sexual/having sex, specify)						
Role playing (specify in notes)						
Other sensation play (specify in notes)						
Other kinky play (specify in notes)						

Below is some free space so you can get creative or fill in what I've missed!

Your Yes, No, Maybe List

Activity	Solo	Giving/partnered	Receiving/partnered	Giving + receiving/partnered	Questions, concerns, notes	✓✓

My Definition of Sex Is . . .

Different strokes for different folks! *Sex* can mean a million different things to a million different people. Though many default to penis-in-vagina penetration as the definition of sex, for many people's bodies and relationship styles, this definition doesn't apply! For some sex can mean mutual orgasm, for some it means the occurrence of any kind of penetration with any kind of toy or body part, and for others sex means an intentional exchange of sexual energy. When it comes to what sex can mean, the possibilities are near endless. So, being clear about your definition of sex to yourself and your partner can help avoid confusion and keep everyone on the same page when answering the question . . . "So, do you want to have sex?"

What's Your Definition of Sex?

The General Vibe of Sex I Like to Create Includes . . .

(Circle all that apply or add your own.)

Sensual	Love-making	Rough	Playful
Funny/silly	Dominant	Submissive	Switchy
Kinky	Tantric	Slow (Take your time . . .)	Rushed (Take me now!)
Quickie	Long, languid session	Creative	Serious
Vocal	Quiet(ish)	Explorative	A way to get off
A way to connect	A way to relax	A way to have babies	A way to inhabit my body
A way to express my affection	A spectator sport	A private affair	

I've Got This Fantasy That . . .

Your brain is a powerful part of your sexual anatomy! Fantasizing can increase pleasure and relaxation and can be fun to share with your partner to utilize for dirty talk or play. If you'd like to share some of your fantasies, jot them down here:

Parts of this fantasy I'd like to try to bring into my real-life sex life include:

Parts of this fantasy that I'd like to keep as fantasy or dirty talk include:

Parts of this fantasy that I'd like to keep to myself include:

Exploring My Maybes
(Don't forget to check the resource guide for some specific exploration suggestions!)

How do you know when a *maybe* has evolved into a *yes* or a *no*? Only you know that for sure in your gut, your mind, and your sexual body, but one way to navigate these edges is by exploring those *maybe*s a little further before jumping in (or out).

A couple of *maybe* activities I've labeled above with a "?" that I'd like to explore further include:

Some ways I'd like to explore these *maybe*s are:
(Circle all that apply.)

Watching relevant porn

Reading relevant erotica

Visiting a sex toy shop

Hiring a sex coach, sex educator, or sex therapist

Attending a play party just to watch and learn

Attending a play party to participate

Attending a sex, sexuality, kink, or relationship conference

Attending a sex, sexuality, kink, or relationship class or
     workshop (online or in-person)

Talking to my therapist about it

Talking to my friend(s) about it

Journaling about it

Finding more info on the subject on social media or online

Trying my *maybe* with myself, by myself

Trying my *maybe* with myself, with a partner present

Trying my *maybe* with my partner with the continued knowledge that we can stop or adjust at any time

Other:

My Verbal Boundaries

How you speak about a person lays a foundational groundwork for their sense of safety, selfhood, and, therefore, potential pleasure in a sexual interaction with you. Happily, a
little word (like using someone's correct pronouns) can go
a long way in laying tracks for a satisfying interpersonal
experience—sexual or otherwise. For more information on
pronouns, gender identity, and what makes language about
both so important, see the resource guide.

My pronouns are:

My gender is:

My sexuality can be defined as:

Other identifiers I'd like you to know about:

During sex, I *love* to be called:

During sex, please *never* call me:

Refer to my sexual anatomy as:

Never refer to my sexual anatomy as:

When it comes to sharing information about the sexy times we have together, I prefer you:
(Check off as many as you want and/or specify.)

☐ Keep me anonymous when talking about it.

☐ I prefer you don't share at all. (I'm very private.)

☐ Only tell close friends.

☐ Ask me before sharing anything.

☐ I'm an open book! Tell whoever and whatever details you want!

☐ Other:

Other verbal boundaries:

My Physical Boundaries

Beyond what's listed in the above sexual activities checklist, here are some other important things to know about my physical boundaries.

Ways I love to be touched outside of sex:

Ways I love to be touched during sex:

Please never touch me this way outside of sex:

Please never touch me this way during sex:

Other physical boundaries:

My Relational Boundaries

I've said it before and I'll say it so many times again: good sex is relational! So, as long as we're talking about sex, let's talk about some relational aspects of sex.

My current relationship status is:

I am currently interested in relationships that can be described as:

(Check all that apply.)

☐ Monogamous
☐ Non-monogamous[3]
    ☐ Polyamorous
    ☐ Solo polyamorous
    ☐ Relationship anarchist
    ☐ Open
    ☐ Open-ish
    ☐ Open to being open
☐ Casually dating
☐ Committed relationship
☐ Friends with benefits (ongoing)
☐ Friends with benefits (occasional)
☐ One-night stand
☐ Long distance
☐ Kinky
☐ Vanilla
☐ Primarily sexual

- ☐ Romantic
- ☐ Aromantic
- ☐ Asexual
- ☐ Interested in long-term planning like marriage, property sharing, or children
- ☐ Other:

Consent Check!

Consent is an active and ongoing process that is mandatory for sex to be mutual, pleasurable, and nonviolent. It's also a practice that can look and sound a little different for every person and in every sexual interaction. Checking in about your particular ways of discussing consent is a proactive step to keep consent thriving in your sex life. Here are a few prompts.

When I'm enthusiastically enjoying sex:

I do:

I say:

I look like:

Signs to check in with me or re-establish consent include when:

I do:

I say:

I look like:

Nonverbal cues that I am *not* into what's going on or have been triggered by something include:

Verbal ways I like to:

Ask for consent:

Give consent:

Deny or revoke consent:

If either one of us *unintentionally* crosses a boundary, here's our plan of next steps. (We'll dive deeper into accidental boundary violations and mistakes in Chapter 10.)

Aftercare and Communication

Aftercare[4] is a term popularized by the BDSM/kink community to refer to the period of time after sex or play during which partners attend to each other's physical, emotional, or psychological needs. Aftercare can be beneficial in all relationships—kinky or not—and can include either casual or involved post-sex caring acts.

Here are a few ideas to get you thinking about how you like to receive care after sharing sex with someone!

Types of Aftercare I'm Interested In
(Check all that apply.)

- Chatting
- Cuddling
- Talking about highlights of the sex we just had
- Side-by-side phone scrolling
- Snacks
- A shower with you
- A shower alone

- Being wrapped in a blanket
- Watching my favorite shows
- Going on a walk
- Other:

Please check in or chat with me:

- Never, I'm good
- The next day
- In three ish days
- Whenever the mood strikes you
- Other:

My favorite communication methods:

- Voice call
- Text
- Social media (here are my handles):
- Email
- In-person hangouts/dates
- Other:

Sexual Health

Talking about sexual health—including your current status of sexually transmitted infections (STIs) and diseases (STDs), your safer-sex and birth control methods, the last time you got tested, and any relevant partner disclosures—can feel intimidating and awkward. This is especially true because we tend to have these conversations with brand-new sexual partners.

However, sexual health conversations are a crucial part of making sure that the sex you're having includes the *informed* consent of all parties involved, and they work toward reducing the cultural stigma around sexual health diagnoses that make these talks so challenging in the first place. Hopefully this section can help break the ice as we all work toward a sexual world where these conversations can be easy as pie.

My last STI/STD screening was on:

My current STI/STD status is:

Safer-sex methods I require:

Safer-sex methods I prefer but don't consider mandatory/ am flexible about:

Birth control methods I require:

Birth control methods I prefer but don't consider mandatory/ am flexible about:

Other notes about my physical, mental, or sexual health that may apply:

Questions I have for my partner about their physical, mental, or sexual health:

Notes to Self

You guessed it, this is a free space.

Other Boundaries:

Important Things to Know about Me:

Questions I'd Like to Be Sure I Ask My Partner:

(For example, "What kind of relationship are you looking for right now?", "Are you on birth control?", "Are you okay with the fact that I'm married but in an open relationship?")

Things on My Mind:

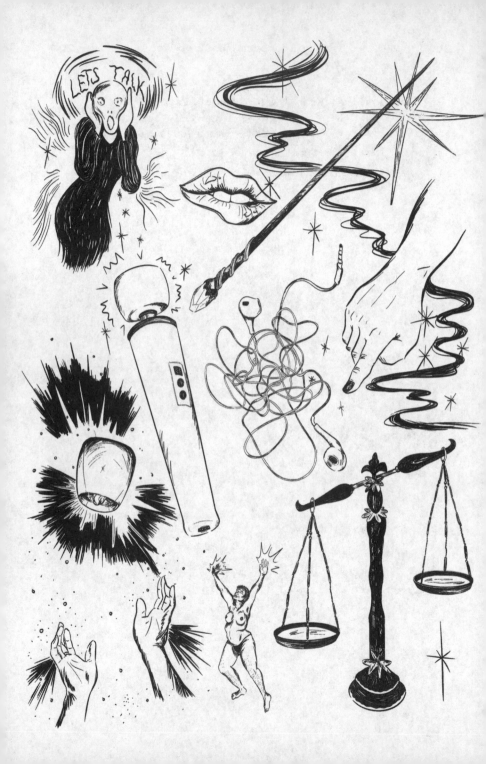

CHAPTER 7

How to Ask for What You Want

Desire is to own the wanting. It is a claim: I want.[1]
—Esther Perel

Rejection is protection.[2]
—Elle Chase, Curvy Girl Sex

Evolutionary Psychology Is Cramping Your Sex Life

When a client comes into my office and tells me, "I don't know how to ask for what I want in bed," they usually don't mean that they literally don't know how to say, "Darling, can you pass the lube?" It's all the fear and anxiety that comes with asking that people need to work through. When a client says, "Help me learn how to ask for what I want in bed," they usually mean one of two things: "I don't know what I want out of sex, so therefore I don't even know what to ask for" (see Chapter 6) and/or "Help me protect myself from abandonment and shame if I ask for something and it doesn't go well." Once clients have done their work in discovering what they want out of sex, they are then, at some point, inevitably faced with actually asking for those wants. The majority of them describe feelings of nervousness, anxiety, or deep fear; fear of embarrassment, rejection, or offending a partner is common, but so is fear of seeming too aggressive, pushy, or demanding.

"Why is it so scary to just ask for what I want!?" I've heard many exclaim. Though a lot of clients feel as though the apparent inability to ask for what they want out of sex is a personal, individual failure, it's actually extremely common, impacted greatly by many of the social-sexual factors we have already covered, and also heavily influenced by our animal nature. Our common relational fears of rejection, disconnection, and judgment are in fact embedded in the evolutionary fears all animals have of threats to their basic survival. These fears come with adaptive automatic responses that help us avoid perceived threats and maximize self-preservation by all means necessary. For us humans, this means that not only are we afraid to ask our partner for what we want in bed for fear of receiving a negative response, but we are also fighting against our historic, evolutionarily hardwired alarm system that's subconsciously blaring the warning "Lion in the bush! Lion in the bush! RUN!" in response to our fear—an automatic response that certainly doesn't make it any easier to introduce our partner to our newfound propensity for latex bodysuits.

Exploring our animalistic roots through evolutionary psychology has given us fascinating perspectives on how we relate to each other, how our practice of monogamy or non-monogamy has evolved,[3] and why and how we are running centuries-old programming when seeking a mate. Evolutionary psychology also has a lot to offer us when exploring the answer to many clients' main question: "Why *is* it so scary to ask for what we want from sex?" The short, dramatic answer is: any threat to our most valued human connection feels like a threat to our very lives.

The long answer is this: as human beings we are, at our core, pack animals. We only survive in relationship to others,[4] we have a tendency for pack behavior and a pack mentality,[5] we find comfort in predictable patterns,[6] and we mitigate our relational risks accordingly. We are wired in our bodies and brains to connect to each other by being viewed as valuable, indispensable, good, and worth keeping around. This is especially true in the context of a romantic or sexual partnership.

During adulthood, a big way we seek and receive survival-based validation and connection is through our sexual relationships (no matter how fleeting or long term the relationship may be). Sex is a big way that we connect to the people we like, love, or simply lust after, so we quickly assess how to maintain that connection once we've made it. Whether we do this by hiding certain parts of our sexual self so as to not scare someone away or making concessions big and small in order to increase our sexual compatibility, we make both intentional and unintentional adjustments to our thoughts, standards, and behaviors in order to maintain a sexual connection. This is especially likely to happen when making a fresh connection in a new, exciting sexual relationship, or when attempting to maintain the stabilizing status quo in a long-term relationship.

Basically, when it comes to sex and relationships, evolutionary psychology subconsciously encourages us to learn quickly how to act so we can stay in the good graces of the pack. This means that, when we consider the possible rupture we could cause in our relational connection by asking for something sexual, we fear we may be shunned or shamed. The asking itself can feel like a huge, scary risk because, evolutionarily speaking, it is.

When our historic, evolutionary systems are alerted to a potential risk to our pack connection, our bodies and minds automatically respond to these perceived external threats using several instinctual survival tools (the most recognizable being popular psychology's fight, flight, freeze, or fawn[7]). One of these survival tools is negativity bias[8] or, basically, the threat-scanner that never rests. Thanks to negativity bias, we are more likely to tune into negative interactions or details, even if they're outnumbered by positive ones. This is responsible for behaviors such as obsessing over the one mean comment on our social media post rather than the 10 compliments. Though negativity bias doesn't really help us out that much here in the modern Twittersphere (hyper-tracking for negative social media comments has been linked to depression and anxiety,[9] for example), it did do us a lot of favors in the past. For example, if a lion were indeed hunting us, our survival mechanisms would go on high alert, making sure that we kept all eyes and ears on that predator, prepping our bodies to fight, run, or play dead. Negativity bias makes sure that we're truly paying attention to that lion rather than kicking back and enjoying the beautiful sunset, getting distracted by a handsome stranger, or doing something that would otherwise get our asses eaten (no, not in the good way).

Our fundamental animal nature continues to automatically function to help us navigate risks to our survival and aid us in our primary evolutionary goal of self-preservation and pack inclusion—good job, evolution! But what does evolutionary psychology have to do with why you're so scared to ask your girlfriend to stick a sex toy up your butt?

Well, when we want to ask our partner to do something during sex, want to divulge a fantasy or a sexual desire, or want to change a well-worn sexual style that we've been doing with our long-term mate for years, our animal instincts are scanning and getting prepared for the risks involved in doing so. If we're getting ready to ask for something and we don't know how it's going to land or what the answer may be (and we rarely do!), we are acutely aware that the answer may be "No! What?!" or something similarly judgmental, rejecting, or connection straining.

We rarely focus on the possibility that our partner may say, "Yes!" or even be super into it themselves. Instead, when we think about asking for what we want out of sex, most of us cannot look away from the risk this ask poses to our connection to our partner (negativity bias at work!). To want fundamentally different things sexually might mean an inevitable conflict, incompatibility, or maybe even a separation, and our evolutionary survival brains simply aren't having that shit. Though it's very, very unlikely that we'll die from sexual incompatibility, our evolutionary survival systems are good at making it seem like we might. We are programmed for relational survival and biologically built to keep our eye out for any potential dangers in the bushes of our sex lives, and for many that means sexual rejection looks a lot like a big ol' scary lion.

Because we are pack animals, we also have a desire to understand and play by the rules, commonly referred to as *pack mentality*. Pack mentality is the pack animal's way of self-regulating their behaviors to be more in line with what is acceptable to or perceived as "normal" behavior within the herd. When you get into an elevator, the unspoken rule is that you face the door.[10] To face backward would be odd and would visually and perhaps relationally, emotionally, and physically separate you from the pack. In the elevator of our collective relationship to sex, you betcha we've got both unspoken ("Don't talk during sex or you'll ruin the [classic] mood!") and spoken ("Pre-marital sex is a sin!!") rules in our pack(s). Some of these rules are excellent for our sex lives ("Practice active consent!") and others, not so much ("Period sex is gross!").

As we saw in Chapter 5 and in Jessa's case specifically, societal expectations and sexual norms influence what we think is okay to ask for, how many asks we're allowed to have, and how we believe our partners will perceive our asks when it comes to sex: "I already asked for another dollop of lube, so requesting another finger is just too much." "She was already game to experiment with handcuffs, so don't push your luck with bringing up your interest in rope bondage." "Your desires are a burden," this same pack-mentality inner voice says, "so stop putting them on your partner already—enough!"

As touched on in the Introduction, mainstream porn and media portrayals of sex have done a great job of artificially pigeonholing people's sexualities along the lines of gender, race, body type, sexual orientation, and so on, which greatly influences our collective perception of what is allowed and normal to desire from sex. For example, women have historically been taught to accept a close-proximity version of what we've asked for sexually (that is, if we drum up the courage to ask in the first place) and are often accused of being rude, emasculating, or slutty if we're too specific or insistent on clarifying our original ask. Men and those who want to exude masculinity, on the other hand, have been largely encouraged to demand or *go get it!* while being discouraged from asking for off-script sexual needs like emotional tenderness, trauma-informed sexual encounters, or certain sex acts like anal sex or sexual domination. Whether you consider yourself to be influenced by traditional gender roles, mainstream porn, conventional media sex scenes, or otherwise rampant sexual lore about what is allowed and who is entitled to what, chances are you've got at least some sense of what is sexually normal along with a societally approved sketch of how to go about getting those desires met, complete with an internal trip wire that'll set off ye olde sexual shame when you begin to trespass the borders of normalcy.

You are totally normal and right in line with your animal instincts if you feel nervous, scared, or uncertain when faced with asking for what you want out of sex. Because of evolutionary psychology, negativity bias, pack mentality, and societal sexual norms, not to mention experiential factors (e.g., that shitty ex that made you feel bad about your kinks), asking for what you want sexually can feel like a *huge* risk. This is true even if it cognitively seems like it should be no big deal. The reality is that the risks we take when we ask for what we want out of sex aren't just immediate (rejection, embarrassment, vulnerability, disconnection), they're also deeply rooted, historically compounded, and psychologically and physically fused to our basic sense of self and survival.

All of this is to say: Asking for what you want from sex can feel like high stakes. And for many good reasons!

Would it help if I told you that there are no lions around here?

Lions and Vibrators and Kinks, Oh My!

The good news is that in your present-day, lion-less bedroom, the stakes of asking for what you want are actually much lower than your evolutionary hardwiring may have you believe. Your perception of the situation may be hijacked by your instinctual need for connection, acceptance, validation, and pack value. And that perception is in your power to shift through questioning your own negativity biases, being selective about which past experiences you allow to dictate your present, and checking in with yourself about the actual stakes of your current situation.

Evolutionary psychology isn't all bad. Learning from patterns, past traumas, and even from our intuitive animal instincts can protect us from making the same mistakes twice, stop us from placing ourselves in harm's way, and help us develop strategies to protect our bodies and emotions. Evolutionarily speaking, this makes perfect sense. If we lived through the horrifying experience of discovering a lion hiding behind a bush, and survived by running away or playing dead, our brain and nervous system will record the details of our successful response so that we have faster access to it for the next time we're under threat. Our efficient evolutionary systems are just looking out for us, asking, "Why not just cut out the middleman? Instead of looking in the bushes to see if there's even a lion there, next time we hear a rustling in the bushes, let's just book it!"

How this evolutionary instinct shows up in your bed might look like this: You had an ex totally kink-shame you when you told them about a fetish, or maybe you had the repeated experience of having your sexual needs ignored or shut down in unproductive ways (running into a lion behind a bush). You may have learned that it's not worth bringing up your kinks to anyone else (running away) or that it's not worth asking for what you want in the first place (playing dead). It's easier, you might learn, to just avoid the topic (don't go anywhere near a bush), shy away from asking your partner(s) questions about what you want (especially if that bush is rustling), or begin to erase those pieces of your sexuality entirely (cutting out the middleman). Though this adaptive strategy is designed by the evolutionarily intelligent system of your brain and body in order to protect you from making the same mistake twice, it's ultimately not that productive in creating your best sex life (unless you're planning on having sex during a safari and truly need to be on the lookout for lions).

Sometimes there are indeed modern-day "lions" hanging out in the bushes of our sex lives, creating an atmosphere that feels less than safe for us. These theoretical sex-life lions can look like trauma history, feeling unsafe with your partner, lack of communication, toxic relationship patterns, and many other thoughts and experiences. Sometimes we're so busy listening for the rustle of a *potential* lion (What if she says no? What if he thinks I'm weird? What if we can never agree on our sex life?) that we haven't even dared to glance at the bushes to see if there actually is a lion there at all—maybe it's just some harmless but rowdy birds, ruining our chances of enjoying the sunset with their menacing-sounding bush-rustling behavior. But we can only know if we look behind the bush, or as the case may be in our sex lives, if we question our own negativity bias and fears, and venture forward in asking for what we want.

If your sexual relationship is fundamentally safe and healthy,[11] it's more likely that the nerves you feel about asking for what you want are more bird than lion. So asking might sound scary or feel familiar to your previous lion-dodging experience, but upon closer examination, your ask or reveal probably isn't actually threatening your survival or connection to your partner as severely as you fear it might. Rather than take nervousness or anxiety as a sure signal that you shouldn't talk about what you want at all, treat these feelings like a check-engine light. Just because the light is on doesn't mean that your car's engine is nearing spontaneous explosion, but it does mean that you should check a couple of things out. Because of our natural negativity bias, most of us will easily come up with a list of things that could possibly go wrong if we ask for what we want in bed (in fact, you probably already have). But if we're to more accurately assess our environment so that we can free up the parts of our brain and bodies that want to bravely receive pleasure, we need to take the time to also ask ourselves, "What could possibly go right?", "Is my survival or connection actually at stake here or are these feelings historical?", and "Am I scared-scared? Or I am nervous-excited?" The worksheet below may help you untangle some of these questions.

My Risky Business

A worksheet to help you assess for lions, birds, and the present-day stakes of your sex life.

When I think about asking my partner for what I truly desire out of sex, I:

Feel:

1.

2.

3.

Think:

1.

2.

3.

Do:

1.

2.

3.

Thanks to these survival strategies for protecting me when:

(Think: Is there a person, situation, experience, relationship, system, or other entity that taught you that you shouldn't ask for what you want [sexually or otherwise] or that it won't go well if you do?)

Turns out, some of my old survival strategies are no longer working for me because:

When asking for what I want out of sex I would *like* to instead:

Feel:

1.

2.

3.

Think:

1.

2.

3.

Do:

1.

2.

3.

I know a partner is safe(r) for me to be sexually vulnerable with when I:

Feel:

1.

2.

3.

Think:

1.

2.

3.

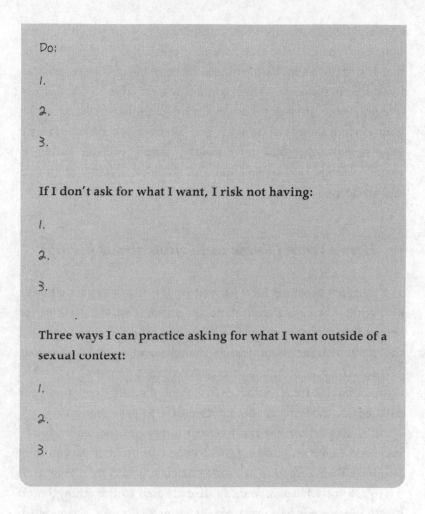

Do:

1.

2.

3.

If I don't ask for what I want, I risk not having:

1.

2.

3.

Three ways I can practice asking for what I want outside of a sexual context:

1.

2.

3.

Without taking the time to examine what your survival signals like fear, nerves, and anxiety are actually pointing to, you may go your entire life catering to imaginary lions. If you do this, you might never allow yourself to feel fully safe or at ease in your sexual interactions, and you'll continue to spend your energy and attention on old patterns. Though these patterns may have been wise and helpful at some point or even key to your survival, these same patterns can also trap you in a present-day sexual routine that is unsatisfying, disingenuous, or straight-up counterproductive to your pleasure. When you are instead able to consciously integrate your past experiences and evolutionary systems with your current (lion-less) context, you can then accurately evaluate your sexual stakes and move toward asking for your authentic sexual pleasure with protection and confidence rather than fear and anxiety.

Here's What I Know to Be True about Asking

The thing about asking for what you want is that it's exactly that—it's asking. Asking is a request, not a demand. Confusing asking for demanding prevents many from creating sexual interactions that they actually want. Asking rather than demanding means that your partner has options. And if your relationship is operating under the assumption that this freedom exists (and it should), know that your partner can and will say yes, no, or maybe to your request.

If your partner has the freedom to say yes, no, or maybe to your asks (more on building this freedom in Chapter 9), you then also have the freedom to ask for as much as you'd like. Your ability to ask for what you want is directly tied to the strength and health of your consent practices, listening skills, and adaptability to the moment. So, if you want to get good at asking, make sure you spend time getting good at your basic relational skills, too.

Sometimes asking leads to rejection, and that's okay. Writer Elle Chase sums it up nice and rhymey: "Rejection is protection."[12] If you ask for what you want, if you venture to set the tone in your sexual interactions, and your (potential) partner scoffs, is a jerk, or even delivers you a very kind and compassionate *no*, you've just gained yourself some valuable information about your potential (in)compatibility as partners. I, for one, do not want to have sex with someone who does not want to have sex with me. Being and feeling genuinely desired is something you deserve to have in your sex life. Molding your desires to fit what you think your partner wants you to want, do, or be, though an understandable pack-mentality instinct, is not actually a clear path to your genuine pleasure.

Asking isn't just ethical and consensual work, it's also efficient work. Asking for what you want and asking your partner what they want really cuts down on the static of the guess-and-test method. Rather than expending all of your energy pulling out antiquated moves from the latest big-name magazine's sex-tips listicles, why not just cut to the chase and literally ask for what truly gets you going, gets you hot, and gets you off? As discussed in Chapter 2, we can obsess over being "good in bed," but if we can't ask our partners what would feel good to them in bed, we'll never really get there. Want to really blow your partner's mind in bed? Ask them how to do it.

Asking doesn't need to start with expertise. You can also ask to just experiment. Yes! You *can* enthusiastically consent to trying something new, even if you're not sure you'll like it because consent means that you can change your mind or make adjustments any time you choose. We don't need to have an exhaustive, perfected, step-by-step guide detailing what we want out of sex, ready to present to our partners in order to have a fulfilling sexual interaction. Co-creating our most pleasurable sex lives is an ongoing practice—a gelatinous thing that we might always be reaching for but never truly, materialistically attain. Instead, the work and the gain is in the art of the practice.

Asking for what you want makes it far more likely that you'll actually get it. Sure, our risk-averse brains and bodies would far prefer that our partners just intuitively know what we want from them but, sorry, that app hasn't been invented yet. It really is up to you to clue your partners in to what it is you want from sex.

Asking is different from desiring. A desire doesn't turn into an ask until you ask for it, if you ask for it at all. Sometimes, desires only appear in your fantasy life and you don't actually want them to appear in your real life and that's totally okay!

You have options when it comes to your desires and what turns you on. You can: 1) fantasize about them privately; 2) share them with a partner on the fantasy level, leaving them available as fodder for things like dirty talk and sexting; 3) convert them into real-life actions that are actually doable in your relationship. (For example, maybe you have a fantasy about having a threesome in outer space. Maybe getting you and two of your adventurous fuck buddies outside the atmosphere isn't attainable, but negotiating a group sex situation in a space-themed Airbnb might be!) Just because something turns you on doesn't mean you want to do it. That's normal and okay! You should ask for the things you actually want, not for *all* of the things you desire (well, unless you want to).

Watch out! Ask and you just might get it. Something sneaky about asking is that you might feel some level of nervousness or anxiety about hearing your partner say, "Yes! I'm super into that!" For example, it might be super hot to think about your bestie having sex with your husband while you watch. But, for some people, when they ask for something like this and their partner says, "Fuck yeah, I wanna do that!" they can be surprised by their complex reactions to getting what they asked for.

This doesn't mean that you've asked for the wrong things, this just means that relationships, sex, and emotions are complicated and that you've hit a new layer of sexual communication: talking about the other asks within your original ask, such as setting boundaries (more to come on boundaries in Chapter 8) and clarifying what you want now that you've got the intel of your emotional reaction to your partner's *yes!* Asking is more like peeling an onion than flipping a light switch—it usually takes more than one move to create your desired outcome.

Asking for what you want starts with giving yourself explicit permission to want what you want. This entire book is devoted to giving yourself permission to discover, communicate about, and experience your genuine desires for a reason: the permission piece is foundationally key to creating your best sex life, and this includes asking for what you want out of that sex life. If giving yourself the explicit permission to want what you want feels too challenging right now, let me help you get started. You inherently have the permission to:

- ★ Ask for more
- ★ Ask for less
- ★ Ask for a break
- ★ Change your mind
- ★ Pause
- ★ Eat a snack, drink some water, use the bathroom
- ★ Be a total pervy kinkster
- ★ Be vanilla
- ★ Be unsure
- ★ Hesitate
- ★ Reevaluate
- ★ Be excited about sex
- ★ Have zero interest in sex
- ★ Like sex

★ Feel weird in your body
★ Feel good in your body

I give myself permission to:
★ _____
★ _____
★ _____
★ _____

Asking is assertive, not aggressive. Make your asks with the understanding that your wanting is not the same thing as getting, expecting, or imposing. Wanting is something you can do whether or not your partner is interested in joining you in exploring the things you want. When done consensually and ethically, asking for what you want is not the same as being an aggressor, a creep, or an inconvenience. Asking is merely a question or suggestion. Your partner always has the permission to say yes, no, or maybe. Give yourself the permission to want, desire, and ask with the understanding that you might not always get it.

How to Ask for What You Want, in Real Life, Now

Evolutionary psychology is interesting and all, but at the end of the day, you still gotta get to the asking part. The process of asking can be broken down into two parts:

1. How do you ask for what you want in general? This might be how you describe your current desires overall such as who you're attracted to (along gender, political, aesthetic descriptors, etc.), what you're into (kink, vanilla, penetra-

tion, cuddles), or what you're emotionally and physically available for (relationships, hook-ups, strictly solo sex). Return to the previous chapter and your Yes/No/Maybe List if you need a refresher on some of your thoughts about these wider-sweeping questions.

2. How do you ask for what you want, in the moment? What kind of directives, requests, boundaries, and edits would you like to make in real time, during your sexual interaction? And perhaps more importantly, how do you do this without being overcome with nerves, anxiety, and hesitation?

Asking for What You Want in General

When we're talking about asking for what you want in general, the line between setting boundaries and asking for something from another person gets a little blurry because setting boundaries and asking for what you desire are two sides of the same coin. You can't really ask for what you want without having your boundaries in place, and you can't put your boundaries in place without knowing what you want or what you do/don't want to ask for—but we'll get more into this in Chapter 8.

Once you've got clarity about your sexual desires, you need to determine which of your desires you actually want to ask for. Just because you're into leather doesn't mean you want to wear leather right this minute, or with your current partner, or necessarily all of the time. Just because you desire something doesn't mean you always want to do it or that you don't have certain criteria about with whom you want to do it with. For example, some people find that wearing a strap-on makes them feel super hot, but only with certain partners. Or, some people love watching porn, but only when they're masturbating alone because it feels too awkward to enjoy with a partner. All of this is normal and you get to determine the lines around your desires and real-world asks in ways that feel best to you, even if that means reserving certain desires for your fantasy realm only.

Let's say that you feel clear about your current desires and what you want to ask for, in general, in your sex and dating life. One way to approach this conversation with another person is to simply tell them about yourself. I find that asking for what you want, in general, is easier when you think of it as sharing your desires and sexual self-knowledge with another person. For example, you could say, "I'm super into leather." This statement is telling your partner about your sexual self. "Is that something you'd be interested in exploring with me?" is making a related, direct ask. Within the framework of sharing information, your self-disclosures and asks are also conveniently doubling as curiosities about the other person and their own boundaries, asks, and limits. Here's one way this could go:

Cam: So, I've been doing a lot of thinking about this and talking about it with my therapist and I've discovered that I am really interested in exploring non-monogamy. I know that this isn't something that we have done before and isn't how our relationship has been structured in the past, so I'm sure you have a lot of questions. But first I'm wondering, is this something you'd be willing to even consider or discuss further with me? Because shifting the structure of our relationship is something I'd like to ask for.

Brit: Wow, I'm feeling pretty surprised by this, to be honest, and it feels like a lot to wrap my head around at the moment. But I'm really glad you're sharing this with me and I'd like to have another day to myself to just sort through my own thoughts and feelings before we come back to this. Overall, though, I am willing to keep talking about it.

Cam: Okay, that's totally understandable. Thank you for being open to the discussion at all. I really love you and also want to be authentic to myself, and this feels really complicated to sort out. I'm glad I don't have to try to sort it out on my own anymore.

If you find yourself about to ask for something in your relationship or sex life that you think your partner(s) may be surprised by, not know a lot about, or have a lot of questions about, it's always a good idea to have a couple (not an overwhelming amount!) of resources to share. For example, a book about nonmonogamy, a social media account dedicated to accurate kink education and information, or a resource that you have personally found helpful. Sharing information and resources can help your partner feel autonomous in getting answers to some of the questions they might have, and it allows the two of you to work on the personal, relational front rather than spending a lot of time and energy on education.

Another thing that many find helpful when faced with asking for what you want in general is one of my favorite therapy hacks: talk about talking about the thing first. As therapists we're trained to spend time with our clients addressing the feelings they have about talking about certain tough topics before they actually talk about the tough topic. This can strengthen therapeutic trust and safety and can also be an important, reflective warm-up for the client before they dive into a challenging story or memory. In a personal, relational context, this can look like talking to your partner about the conversation you want to have before initiating the actual conversation itself.

If it feels insurmountable, or if you feel too vulnerable, to jump right into the tough topic, zoom out a little bit and first have a chat with your partner about the anxieties and hesitations you have about having a conversation about the topic. This can be done about a specific talk you want to have ("I want to talk about the structure of our relationship, but I'm feeling really scared to rock the boat with you") or it can be done about a general genre of talks ("I want to start talking about our sex life more, but every time I think about doing it, I just get super nervous and shut down"). Talking about talking can help break the ice, lower the stakes, and can enlist your partner's help in facilitating these nerve-wracking conversations together as collaborators. Here's how this might look:

Trevor: Hey, can I get your help with something? It's about our relationship.

Noel: Of course, babe, lay it on me.

Trevor: Well, I've been thinking that I really want to start exploring new things in our sex life. But, every time we're making out and things seem to be going in that direction I just get all weird and locked up and just don't say anything new!

Noel: Oh, okay. I mean, are you okay with the sex we are having?

Trevor: Oh, for sure! I think our go-to sex routine is really satisfying and I'm definitely present and consenting. I just want to mix things up, but I just feel *so* nervous about it.

Noel: Okay, yeah that makes sense to me. I want to learn new things about you and myself as a sexual person, too. Do you think it would take some of the nerves out of the situation if instead of bringing new stuff up during sex we make a coffee date and talk about some of this stuff before we find ourselves back in bed together?

Trevor: Yeah, actually, that seems like a great idea. I feel less nervous already.

Noel: Good! Let's get something in the calendar. This is exciting!

And here's a short-and-sweet version of how talking about talking about the thing might happen in a more casual, dating context rather than an established relationship, pulled from my very own, real-life experience:

Me, in my twenties, pulling up to the house of a dude who I've been on a couple of very casual dates with but now things are about to heat up, booty-call style. Texting him from his driveway:

Me: Hey, I'm outside.

Him: Okay. Are you . . . going to come in?

Me: . . .

Me: . . . Yes. Listen, I haven't actually slept with a new person in quite a while and I'm nervous.

Him: Oh, I'm totally nervous, too. But I think it's gonna be great.

Me: Really? Okay, that makes me feel better. I want to talk about what we're actually going to do together before we do it, but I feel like a cheesy dork about it.

Him: No, you're not a cheesy dork! I mean, you are, but we should totally talk about that stuff first. I'm down.

Me: Okay.

Him: Do you want to come in to do that though . . . or are you just gonna keep texting me from my driveway?

Me: LOL. I'll come in.

Of course, there are many ways conversations about desire, fantasies, and general asks can be broached. Finding the way that's a good fit for you and your partner(s) is important because conversations about desires will be ongoing as your desires shift and change. What you thought was just a fantasy might be something you actually want to ask for, what was once a turn-on might suddenly become a turn-off, or you might have new asks to bring to your relational table. Here are some other ways you might ask for what you want in general, also known as sharing information about your desires and sexual self with another person:

- State your desires up front on dating apps such as "Experienced in and interested in consensual kink and seeking others who are the same" or "Looking to date people available for LTRs only."
- Broach the conversation over text if bringing up your ask in person is too nerve-wracking. However, continue the conversation in person to avoid misunderstandings and to keep best consent practices intact.
- Share the fantasy you were just playing with in your mind during sex with your partner once sex is over, such as, "I just had the best fantasy while we were having sex. Can I tell you about it?" and then ask them if they want to share any of theirs with you. Remember, clarify what you are and are not interested in trying in real life.
- Ask the question "Is there anything you want to do differently or anything new you want to do in our sex life?"

as a conversation starter about boundaries and desires with your partner.

- Talk about your desires and what you want out of sex in the chatbox of your current dating app before you and a match decide to meet up for dating, sex, or both so that some of these basic foundations are already set ahead of time. Don't forget to ask them about their desires and asks, too.
- Bring your new sexual or relational ask up in your next couples therapy appointment so that a professional can help mediate the discussion and clarify any potential miscommunications.
- Gift your lovers, partners, and even friends a copy of this book.

Ultimately, these tips to asking for what you want in general are great ways to kickstart the conversation about new things you want to explore, things you've always been curious about but still feel hesitation around, and any changes or updates that you'd like to make to your current sex life or relationship. When these conversations go well (we'll get into when they don't go well in Chapters 9, 10, and 11), they also lead to learning new things about your partner and their desires, limits, and boundaries while creating open space for them to make asks as well.

Asking for What You Want in the Moment

Asking for what you want out of sex, during the actual act of sex itself, is a different animal entirely. Clothes are off, adrenaline is high, dopamine is flowing,[13] and interactions are happening in real time. Basically, all of the barriers that may be popping up in your sex life that we've discussed in this book so far—evolutionarily psychological lions, negativity bias, unhelpful social messages about sex, your positive and negative personal experiences, your automatic thoughts, your Pleasure Pessimism, and sexual imposter syndrome—are being paired with the awesome and enjoyable elements of sex, like touch, fantasy, orgasm, pleasure, connection, euphoria, love, affection, excitement, thrill, and affirmation—and it's all happening within the real, time-based confines of a sexual experience. To top things off, this sexual experience is happening with another person (or people) having their own individual perspective of this experience, complete with all of the same barriers and benefits of sex, at the same time, in the same moment. Fucking *phew*! And in the midst of all this, you're supposed to gather your wits about you enough to ask for what you want in the moment? If you really want to have the kind of sex you really want to have then, yes, you sure are.

Besides, "Well then, you better think fast!" I've got some other, more helpful advice on how to conjure your focus to do just this.

Do your homework before the sex even starts. We don't have a plethora of available examples of how to ask for what you want during sex. It's not often modeled in porn, media, or by (all of) our real-world partners. This means we've got to practice how to ask for what we want and how to give directives to our (willing and consenting) partners.

Remember that PB&J activity from grade school where you had to give detailed instructions to your teammate about how to make a PB&J and they had to follow your instructions word-for-word, so that if you gave shitty directions (like forgetting to tell them to take the bread out of the bag first) then it was a hilarious portrayal of the importance of clear communication? (Or is this activity no longer available in our gluten-free, peanut-allergic classrooms?) Well, your ideal cunnilingus experience is your PB&J, and your partner might need detailed instructions on how to make that snack to your precise preferences. Do you know how to describe the kind of sex acts and stimulation you want? Do you know your own anatomy? Are you familiar with your own plea-sure? Get there first so that you can help someone else understand how you tick. Write it out for yourself or practice in the mirror first if you have to. The resource guide at the back of this book may aid in this important mission, too.

Start with one word and build from there. Asking for what you want with ease and confidence is something that happens with practice, not overnight. A great way to practice the art of the ask is by starting with one-word directives like *slower* or *lower*. This can help you get used to using your voice during sex and can feel like a safe way to test the waters of how your partner receives directions. Remember, if consent is thriving in your relationship, your partner will follow your directives because they genuinely want to, which also helps you feel more free and able to ask for these things in the first place.

Show and tell. When it comes to asking for what you want during sex, sometimes words alone are not going to cut it. Body language cues and physical instructions like taking your lover's hand and moving it just where and how you like it are all sexy ways to show them what you want. However, make sure to pair these physical components with verbal components, as bodily hints alone aren't clear enough to get your ask across or to help your partner truly understand what you're asking for. In general, when it comes to sex, body language alone is never a complete communication, but it can definitely help.

Ask first to set the example and the tone. Don't forget, you're not the only one in this sexual interaction who has wants, needs, desires, and perhaps a healthy dose of asking anxiety. Create more space for asking to be part of your sexual interaction by asking your partner what it is they want you to do: check in mid–sex act with questions like, "Is this how you want me to touch you?" or tell them, "I want to know exactly how to make you feel good, so don't hesitate to tell me what to do." Not only does this open the door to your partner's asking comfort but it can normalize asking in general so that you're freer to make asks, too.

Commit to five seconds of bravery. Not even minutes— seconds. In Chapter 5, we talked about the power of acting with five minutes of bravery, in the spirit of Ralph Waldo Emerson. But when it comes to asking for what you want out of sex, during sex, sometimes all it takes is a mere five seconds of bravery to spit out a short ask like, "Can you shift your hip to the left?" Remember, undoing limiting Negative Narratives and Pleasure Pessimism is done little by little as we gradually disprove our fears over time. Taking five seconds of bravery to say a few words about what you want and then having those words received well can actually be very powerful in the big picture of asking for what you want out of sex.

Talk about talking about the thing. Yep, this little therapist hack can work here, too. If you want to start making more asks in your sex life but feel awkward about how to do this, then talk about exactly that, first.

Fold asks into dirty talk. Sometimes asks can look like clinical discussions complete with an open educational manual, like it did when I was rediscovering my G-spot (Chapter 3), and sometimes asks can just be straight-up hot to hear. For example, "I want you to get on your knees and do exactly what I tell you to do for the next fifteen minutes" or "Can you sneak up behind me in the shower like you did that one time in Miami and take me right there under the showerhead?" Of course, these kinds of dirty-talk asks only work when you and your partner have an established dynamic complete with consent practices that make these kinds of asks possible by keeping them optional, well-boundaried, and mutually understood. Whispering your ask in your partner's ear like a sweet nothing can be a great way to communicate if this type of communication is already a clear and consensual part of your relationship.

Make a compliment sandwich. No, not more PB&J, but another school-days-inspired sex-life tip—sandwich your ask between a couple of compliments. For example, "Your mouth feels so good right now. Can you do softer circles with your tongue? Ooh, yes, just like that." This can be a hot ego boost for your partner as well as a great segue into asking for what you want in the moment.

Own your ask. Whether it's from guilt, shame, or other negative experiences, some people feel the need to apologize for their wants or overexplain why they're asking for what they're asking for. To those people I want to say: There's no need to do this. It's totally fine for you to want harder penetration, to want to use your vibrator to get off, to need an extra pillow under your hips, or to want those handcuffs to squeeze you a little tighter. The more you can bring confidence to the things you want and ask for them without shame or hesitation, the easier it will be for your partner to respond without their own shame or hesitation rising to surface. The more you're able to do the groundwork to truly feel deserving of your desires and pleasure, the easier asking will be.

Grant yourself an unlimited supply of communications. Your most pleasurable sex can only happen with your full participation in communicating what that pleasure looks like for you. Actually getting what you asked for is usually not a one-liner event. (Remember: onion, not light switch.) You'll need to use more than one sentence to clarify what you want, correct a misunderstood directive, or make further adjustments to the sexual experience. By allowing yourself unlimited communications, you resist limiting your sexual self and you also give your partners ample opportunity to truly understand and satisfy you.

Getting Comfortable with Asking

I'm a relatively visible sex columnist situated in a cluster of small, progressive, liberal towns. There's a little cartoon of my face next to my weekly column in the local, free alternative newspaper. The column often leads people to my Instagram, which contains curated details about my life, my dog, my Shibari rope hobby, my latest endorsement of the newest sex toy to cross my desk (bed), and my double-tappable advice about sex and relationships. More often than not, new clients come into my office with at least some predetermined thoughts or impressions about me and my relationship to my own sex life. Sort of like Lincoln from Chapter 1, but in a far more professional setting and atop only slightly sturdier Ikea furniture.

While other therapists (and clients of other therapists) have told me of their awkward struggles to navigate how and when to bring up the topic of sex, within 15 minutes, I typically have new clients talking to me about buttplugs, orgasm woes, and their latest trip to the dungeon. I also get comments like, "I know this probably sounds stupid to someone like you, but I could never talk to my partner about that," "You're obviously like some kind of superpowered rarity who just doesn't fall prey to sexual stigma and shame," and "I'm here to learn how you do it; how did you get to be so comfortable talking about sex?"

I get it. I certainly seem like someone who is good at the asking. But the reality is I am not immune to sexual stigma and shame (is anyone?), and even if I am good at asking for what I want out of sex, who says I'm *comfortable*? Asking for what you want is hard for everyone.

But know this: you can absolutely have a stellar, pleasure-explosion of a sex life chock-full of consent, communication, and self-work and still be like, "Did he actually like that or is he just being gracious?", "I can't believe I said that during sex, she must think I'm so weird!", "I wonder what my butthole looks like right now" (answer: probably like a butthole), or "He'd do anything for love, but he probably won't do *that*" (as you should know by now, you won't know until you ask). You can absolutely start to practice asking for what you want out of sex *before* it feels completely easy, comfortable, and natural to you. In fact, this kind of practice is exactly how the majority of us (even the sex therapists amongst us) will learn how to ask for what we want.

Giving yourself permission to talk about sex and what you want out of it isn't superpowered into you via some kind of mutant sex-positive spider bite (though, I would definitely watch that movie). Finding comfort in your sexuality isn't a one-time factory installation that you missed out on and now can never get. Knowing what you want out of sex and giving yourself permission to ask for it is a skill that you can develop and practice, starting immediately.

Asking for what you want out of your sex life is something most of us need to do on purpose—not once shame is removed but because you know how to manage that shame, not because asking is easy but because you're willing to be brave in your asks, and not because you were handed this skill but because you did the work on yourself and in your relationships to build it.

Here in this book, we talk a lot about developing helpful, concrete skills; however, there is actually no step-by-step recipe to follow in creating sexual comfort in your life. Your sexual evolution will look different from your partner(s)', your friends', and mine. Becoming confident in your desires, your sexuality, and in your sexual communication certainly does not mean that you will always feel cushy, comfortable, certain, or self-assured. I know I'm not! My body still does things during sex I wish it wouldn't, and every now and then I still think, "I wonder what my butthole looks like right now" (answer: still, probably like a butthole). I don't think *anyone* is existing in their sex life feeling zero anxiety/shame and 100 percent comfortable/confident. So, if you're waiting to feel that way or stalling until your own sex-positive spider comes up and bites ya, you're going to be waiting for much longer than you'd probably like to.

Shift your goal away from feeling 100 percent brave, easy, and comfortable, and toward feeling slightly less shame, slightly more confident in your desires, and slightly braver in your asks. Then, keep progressively moving those bars in the right direction until the skills it takes to move them become familiar. Your sex life will always be changing and evolving. Therefore, the aim here isn't to create a perfect sex life and then freeze it in time. The aim is to get good at keeping up with the evolution of your and your partners' desires. In order to do this, you need to sharpen the skills it takes to ask for what you want out of sex, not wait for them to be delivered to you. Because ultimately, if you want to have a long and satisfying sex life, for your whole life, you're going to have to ask for what you want more than once.

I Don't Want to Be a Creep
10 Tips to Asking for What You Want from Sex without the Ick Factor

"How do I ask for what I want out of sex, dating, and relationships without coming off like a total creep?" This is an oft-cited concern I hear from both clients and friends when they're thinking about asking someone out, bringing up a new desire with an established partner, or introducing a new partner to their turn-ons.

While it's great to strive to not be sexually creepy, usually the people voicing these worries: a) aren't typically creeps by very nature of the fact that they're thinking actively about how they're coming off to other people when talking about sex, and b) seem to mistakenly think that voicing their desires = guaranteed "creepiness," which is certainly not an absolute or accurate equation.

As both a sex-advice professional and a longtime recipient of both creepy and not creepy conversations about desire and sex, here are some lines to draw when wondering to yourself, "Am I being creepy?"

1. First, a reminder: it's okay to have desires. Having and verbalizing your desires does not inherently make you creepy. *How* you state your desires, on the other hand, might.

2. Creepy is unaware and imposing. What often feels creepy about a sexual ask or share is the sense that something is being left unsaid or unchecked. If you want to talk about your

desire, do it. Don't obscure portions of what you want to do, or otherwise manipulate your language to mislead your sexual partner. Though the phrase "Netflix and chill" isn't necessarily creepy (depending on who says it, what their relationship is to you, and how), it is a great example of a sexual ask that aims to obscure what the actual ask is.

3. Resist the creep by knowing and sharing your intentions, wants, limitations, and boundaries. When talking about your desires, do so in a well-rounded way. What do you want to do? How do you want to do it? What are your concerns or limits? Showing that you've put active thought into what you want and voicing any personal hesitations (this is especially true for kinks) demonstrates that you are a trustworthy and thoughtful human being, not just someone belligerently looking to get what they want.

4. Know yourself and own it. Do your own work to explore your desires and unpack any shame you hold on your side of things so that it doesn't (creepily) leak onto others or seep into the interaction. If you're holding on to sexuality-based self-loathing, inner criticism, or disgust, it'll likely show up in your sexual interactions, whether you intend it to or not. Though I'm not saying you have to be 100 percent shame-free in order to avoid creep status, if you're completely unaware of your own hang-ups, this unacknowledged part of you can come out as undesirable behaviors like shaming the other person, aggressive come-ons, detachment from yourself, or other actions that definitely have an ick factor, especially in a sexual context.

5. Be clear and brave. Watering down your actual desire (e.g., asking, "Do you want to hang out?" rather than directly asking, "Do you want to go on a date with me sometime?") can feel like a creepy bait and switch. Imagine showing up to an acquaintance's house expecting a platonic board game night and coming in to a three-course candlelit meal on the table.

6. Look for and check in with nonverbal or socially polite cues. Many people have been socially indoctrinated to say *yes* or to file down a clear *no* to an easier-to-swallow *maybe* in response to unwanted invitations. If you ask someone for something or disclose a desire to them, and they seem to have shutdown body language or voice an unclear response, check in, clarify, or just plain back off and let them approach you about the topic at their own pace at a later time (if they want to approach you at all).

7. Leave breathing room—physically, mentally, and logistically. When you broach the topic of a new desire or make an ask, do so in an appropriate context. If you don't really know the person, give them physical distance when asking them out rather than standing over them. If you've got an established relationship, bring up new sexual ideas while you're cuddling or having dinner, not when you're literally in the middle of having sex. Then, allow the person adequate time and space to think about your ask or clarify what you're asking. Don't apply pressure, pout, or rush them.

8. Do not make demands. Don't make an ask until you feel confident that you can accept *yes*, *no*, and *maybe* without react-

ing in a way that would pressure the person to conform to your ask or give you a disingenuous answer. Demands can sound like, "If you really loved me, you would XYZ" and "Way to give me blue balls." (Guess what? Blue balls isn't real.).

9. Revisit asks with care and consent. Depending on the nature of your relationship with the person in question, it can be totally appropriate to revisit a desire discrepancy (more on mismatched sexual desires in Chapter 11) or a boundary incompatibility. However, do this carefully to avoid being creepy. Ask the other person if there's a good time to revisit the topic at hand and don't make it your goal for the other person to shift their boundaries to better accommodate yours. Conversely, asking about the status of a *no* boundary relentlessly is not cool.

10. Creepy is in the eye of the beholder. Something you feel certain isn't creepy may totally creep someone out. Or maybe one person will be totally welcoming of your approach and the next person won't feel comfortable with it at all. If someone tells you they're uncomfortable with the way you're talking about sex with them, accept the feedback, respect their boundaries, problem solve when appropriate, and be gentle with yourself and others as we all travel along the learning curve of becoming well-rounded sexual human beings in a largely sex-negative and misinformed society.

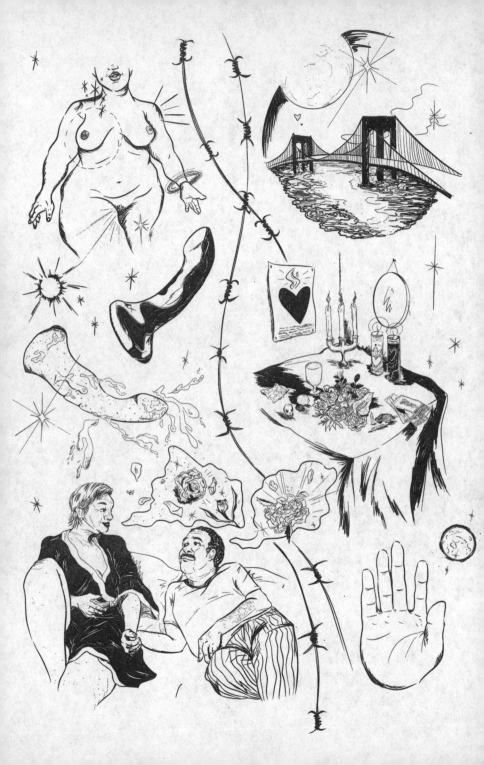

CHAPTER 8

Setting Your Sexual Boundaries

Daring to set boundaries is about having the courage to love ourselves, even when we risk disappointing others.[1]
—Brené Brown

The best sex is "Fuck Yes" sex.[2]
—Mark Manson

My new client Jack says, "Okay, this is probably going to sound weird."

How many times has one of my clients started a sentence in this way (while looking out the window next to my office chair, at the pattern in the carpet by their feet, at the semi-alive plant in the corner, anywhere but at my face)?

Me: People literally come into my office to tell me their sexual secrets—all day. Best-case scenario, I'll just be impressed if you manage to weird me out.

Jack, letting out a little laugh: Okay, I don't like getting blow jobs.

Me, very much not weirded out: Why is that weird?

Jack: I don't know, because all dudes are supposed to like blow jobs?

Me: You don't and you're a dude.

Jack: Well, yeah but that's what I'm saying, I think that's weird. Isn't that weird? Like what is wrong with me?

Me: I can think of at least three dudes off the top of my head who don't like blow jobs and I'm just one person in the world. But that's not really the point—why don't *you* like blow jobs?

Jack: They just really freak me out. They make me nervous, I can't relax, anytime a new person tries to go down on me I just, like, shut down, and then I don't know what to do—I'm like damaged in some way or something.

Me: Yeah, I mean it sounds like blow jobs definitely don't feel good to you, so it makes sense to me that you wouldn't like them. But so what? Why does it matter to *you* that you don't like blow jobs?

Jack: Well, that's why I'm here. I went on a Tinder date last month and she was giving me a blow job and seemed super into it and, I don't know, I just like freaked out. I ended the hook-up and made up some excuse about why I needed to leave but it was totally obvious that something weird was up with me. It was so fucking awkward. And then she texted me a few days later and told me that she was getting back together with her ex and so couldn't go out with me again.

Me: Maybe she got back together with her ex.

Jack: I don't think she did. I think I weirded her out, with the blow job thing. And now I'm scared to hook up with a new person, because what if it happens again?

Me: Do you think it would be possible to tell a new date that you don't like getting head and would rather do other things?

Jack: Ugh, I just don't even want to have to *have* that conversation. I just want to stop being a weirdo and enjoy getting my dick sucked like everybody else!

Me, laughing: Alright then. Well, we can definitely do some work around why you feel like you don't like blow jobs, and whether or not we can figure out how you might find a way to like them, but I'm also curious about why it seems so scary to you to tell a partner what you don't like. Even if it changes down the line, right now the truth is that you don't like blow jobs. But, for many people, blow jobs can be part of a sexual experience so it might come up. So, it might be worth figuring out what to do if/when it does, right?

Jack: Yeah, that makes sense.

Over the next six months of regular therapeutic sessions together, Jack and I talk a lot about blow jobs. Well, sort of. Mostly we talk about his relationship to blow jobs—how his mental, emotional, and physical responses to them come from earlier negative sexual experiences, how our bodies can trap this kind of trauma (whether big or small) and record it in an attempt to protect us from a recurrence of a traumatic event,[3] and how up until now he's never been able to see his aversion to this specific sexual act as valid, okay, or understandable. We talk about how this has been further impacted by societal messaging that "dudes don't experience sexual traumas," which, not so coincidentally, has also contributed to his core belief that "all dudes love getting their dicks sucked" (spoiler alert: they don't) and that he's somehow broken (spoiler alert #2: he isn't).

Gradually, we work on some things: 1) that this core belief isn't the absolute truth (not all dudes love getting their dicks sucked!); 2) how this core belief has hurt his internalized perception of himself as a sexual partner ("broken," "weird," and "damaged"); 3) how undoing these beliefs about himself and others can make more space for him to share his authentic sexual self with his partners by telling them his boundaries—without shame, fear, or second-guessing himself; and 4) we agree that a sexual partner who automatically rejects anyone because they have a boundary isn't a sexual partner you really want to get sexual with, anyway.

Not to toot the horn of collaborative therapeutic work, but this very effectively changes Jack's sex life.

As with most topics discussed in therapy, things are much easier said than done. Boundary work in particular is deeply challenging work. However, it's worthwhile work because along with setting strong sexual boundaries comes, in the words of *The Subtle Art of Not Giving a Fuck*'s author, Mark Manson, much more "'Fuck Yes' sex."

I've found that most people have misunderstood the word *boundaries* as defined *only* by the act of telling people what they can't do. In reality, we can't have *yes* without *no*, or *no* without *yes*. There are two sides to the coins of our boundaries, and one fails to exist without the other. Saying "No," "Not there," "Not like that," or even "Not ever" leads us to our "Yes," "Fuck yes," "Do not ever stop doing exactly that except for maybe slightly more pressure—*yes!*" Boundaries include saying "No" and also include:

1. Creating space for *yes* by delineating the lines around that space, and
2. Sharing information about yourself and your sexual desires.

Whether it's your feelings about blow jobs, a non-monogamous agreement, that new thing you want to try in bed, or how/when to introduce your new partner to your favorite vibrator, the opportunities to state your boundaries are an ever-present, necessary part of all consensual sexual relationships, and you've probably been setting plenty of boundaries without even realizing it ("I'm too tired," "I've got a headache," "Use a condom"). However, from what I've observed, the most thriving sexual relationships include *intentionally* setting boundaries—with confidence, directness, honesty, and regularity. Setting our boundaries is what actually sets the stage for our best sex lives, and yet, rarely do we talk about them as directly as we should. We're going to change that.

What Are My Sexual Boundaries, Anyway?

Sexual boundaries are the container you create around yourself that holds your sexual pleasure in the safest and most comfortable way possible. You could imagine this as a fence in a field or a vase holding water. Personally, when I think about sexual boundaries, I think of each *yes*, *no*, and *maybe* as an individual brick, building a path toward what I really want out of a sexual interaction. In this way, I can see my boundaries as firm yet gentle, handled individually and with care, and as a guide for my partners rather than as a wall between us.

Sexual boundaries control who has access to you, when, and how. Sexual boundaries exist around your body, of course, but they also exist around your mind, your emotions, your sexual energy, your fantasies, and even around who gets to know where you stash your sex toys. Thanks to the Yes/No/Maybe List in Chapter 6, you've got a great start on defining your sexual boundaries. But for a little refresher, sexual boundaries can include (among many, many other considerations):

- How you do/don't like being touched
- How you define sex and what it means to you
- How you do/don't want to be talked about (such as labels for your body parts, gendered language, and even dirty talk)
- Which sex toys you want to use, with whom, and how
- Whether or not you're open to a second date
- What you like to do after sex (and/or during aftercare) like cuddling, eating a snack, taking a shower, or even having some alone time to decompress
- Which sex acts you're open to—those you love, hate, feel *meh* about, or are still figuring out
- Your birth control method and/or your personal stance on abortion, pregnancy, and childbirth
- Whether you're open to monogamy, non-monogamy, or somewhere in between
- What kind of kinky dynamic you're into, if any at all
- How you do or don't want to define the relationship
- The "flavor" of sex you're looking for (rough, romantic, quick, sensual, spiritual, etc.)
- Who you do/don't want to have sex with
- If you want to have sex at all—now or ever
- How you define your sexuality, your gender, or your relationship style
- Which lube brand you prefer

Unfortunately, a common first way we get acquainted with our boundaries is when a boundary is either crossed or closely toed. While anger, hurt (emotional or physical), or even mild annoyance can all be unpleasant feelings, they are strong indicators that a boundary has been too closely approached or violated entirely. Often, strong emotions or uncomfortable physical sensations can precede awareness or insight about what, exactly, has caused them. If such emotions come up after a hook-up, during sex, mid-masturbation, or even just hearing about someone else's sexual experiences or watching a sex scene in a movie, this is a great time to stop or pause and, once the flurry of feelings has settled, check in with yourself and get curious.

A client, let's call her Kira, once hired a pro-domme for a kinky flogging session after becoming curious about this kink but not yet wanting to bring it into her personal dating life with people she might later see in the neighborhood coffee shop. Mid-flogging session, the pro-domme accidentally and lightly whomped Kira in the back of the head with the flogger rather than entirely on her back as her aim intended. Kira, who had done her research and knew this was a safety concern, noticed that she was unable to re-lax into their kinky play and instead became hypervigilant about safety, worried about the pro-domme's actual expertise, and an-noyed that she was now paying a professional to do a less than-professional job. She paused the session using their previously agreed-upon safe word and let her know that her aim had missed and needed to be improved moving forward. The pro-domme, having not realized, thanked her for speaking up, and their play continued without further error. As they continued their explo-ration, Kira was far more relaxed and, just as importantly, felt empowered by her own reinforcement of a boundary. Moving for-ward into her new, kinkier sex life with non-professional dates, Kira now knew that taking extra time to discuss the importance of skill level and basic safety was an important part of her bound-aries discussions with future partners and, having practiced this boundary setting in the context of a professional session, she felt more confident in her ability to set and adjust her boundaries as needed in the future.

But we don't always need to wait for the hot stovetop to burn us (or the pro-domme to whomp us in the head) before we realize that we shouldn't touch it. Solid, proactive sexual boundaries start with solid, proactive sexual self-exploration. The Yes/No/ Maybe List in Chapter 6 is an excellent tool to utilize here, but so is masturbation, fantasy, journaling, reading a book about sex,[4] or even just thinking about your sex life while waiting in line: "What limits do I want to set in order to feel safer, happier, and more turned on during sex?", "What do I want to ask for?", "How do I want to ask for it?"

If these answers seem hard to grasp, reverse engineer your boundaries by starting with assessing what your sexual and relational needs might be. The nonviolent communication movement is known for circulating handy lists[5] of relational and personal needs that all human beings might consider necessary to their happiness, comfort, and connection with others. Exploring one of these lists can help put into concrete words what you might be seeking from a sexual connection such as *joy*, *love*, *creativity*, and *acceptance*. Once you have a fuller picture of your needs, think about what boundaries or limits you might want to set in order to create the conditions for you to get these needs met in a sexual context. For example, if you're LGBTQQIA+-identified and need acceptance, you might set some boundaries around who you're looking to hook up with based on political leanings or belief systems. If you need love from a sexual connection, you might have a boundary around how well you'd like to know someone before getting sexual with them, or you might choose to wait until you feel a certain emotional connection. If you need safety, like my flogging-exploring client, you might have boundaries in place concerning what kind of riskier activities you're willing to do and with whom, and how you'd like to determine who would make a safe kinky playmate.

Not knowing can trigger anxiety in most of us. This anxiety can also trick us into thinking that if we don't know everything about something, we can't set limits around it. But this isn't entirely true. Sometimes we will have a clear picture of our boundaries before we head into a sexual space. Sometimes we will learn a new boundary during sex. And, usually for most of us, identifying and setting our boundaries will be an ongoing, cumulative self-discovery process.

Your Sexual Self-Worth

Setting good sexual boundaries starts with giving a shit about yourself—your body, your pleasure, your orgasm, your shared experience with your sexual partners, and the limits inherent in all of these things. Feeling confident that your sexual boundaries are valid and important is the first step to drawing lines around what you find precious (yourself! your sex life! your experience!) with confidence and ease. Wanting to take the inherent risk in setting a limit (saying "No," "Not there," "Not like that," or "Not ever") is most powerfully motivated by knowing that you absolutely deserve and are entitled to your most pleasurable sexuality. These things can be tricky to truly know because it's not often that we're raised to believe that our unique sexual desires and limits are perfectly valid. So, I'm here to tell you: as long as consent and safety are intact, *your sexual desires and limits are perfectly valid.*

In Jack's case, his culturally sanctioned beliefs that "all dudes love blow jobs," "men don't experience sexual traumas," and "men don't get emotionally triggered during sex" led him to having difficulty confidently setting a boundary around the specific sex act of blow jobs. His fear was that doing so would somehow confirm that he is "weird" or "broken" for even having such a boundary in the first place. This, in turn, led Jack to sexual shame and its beloved companion, silence.

If and when your desires lay outside of "acceptable" sexual boundaries (such as being kinky, non-monogamous, liking sex toys, certain sex positions or acts, or even just liking sex in general), it can feel like your sexual experiences aren't entitled to boundaries at all, as if hopping one fence makes all others meaningless, leaving you to run through an open, infinite field of sexual freakdom. Sure, sounds fun on some level, but also sounds like a great way to have no idea where you're going or how to guide your sexual partner to get there with you.

Other people may have repeated experiences of their boundaries being violated despite setting them clearly, and still others who have found themselves in a context of sexual violence, assault, or trauma may believe that setting boundaries is a pointless project. When your lived experience (especially when repeated) of setting your limits has not paid off in the direction of pleasure, it can be even harder to believe that setting your boundaries is worthy work. First, you are absolutely not alone and I'm sorry that the inability of other people to listen and respect your boundaries, limits, and the basics of consent have reinforced this negative messaging and have, ultimately, made your work harder here. I hope that I'm not the first or last person to tell you: your boundaries are a human right and you are worth the energy it takes to discover, assert, and protect them. For further reading and information on working through sexual assault, traumas, and triggers, please see the resource guide.

Boundaries aren't something you earn by proving your personal or sexual worth. As a person, you are inherently entitled to them, and setting them is a gift to your partners and yourself.

While a lack of boundaries can masquerade as being low-key, edgy, low-maintenance, or, in Jack's case, normally masculine, not setting any limits around yourself or your sexual interactions is actually disorienting and anxiety-provoking for most sexual partners and disrespectful to your sexual self. By not drawing bold lines around our sexual desires, we keep things vague and minimize their importance to ourselves and our partners. Instead, we should mark our sexual maps with bright colors, clear directions, and visible limits.

Again, when it comes to boundaries, there are two sides of the coin, impossible to separate from one another: Every time you say *no* to something, you are opening up space for and saying *yes* to something else. Without saying *no*, you'll likely never find your genuine sexual *yes*.

Worksheet: My No/Yes Coins

Think about some limits you have in your sexual relationship (either with yourself or others). What are you saying *yes* to by way of setting that limit?

Jack's example: When I say "No" to <u>receiving oral sex</u> // I say "Yes" to <u>being less anxious and having more enjoyable hook-ups</u>.

Kira's example: When I say "No" to <u>non-kinky partners</u> // I say "Yes" to <u>sex I'm actually into rather than the sex I was having with my ex-husband</u>.

When I say "No" to _____ //
I say "Yes" to _____ .

When I say "No" to _____ //
I say "Yes" to _____ .

When I say "No" to _____ //
I say "Yes" to _____ .

Think about some aspects of your sexual self or your sex life that you'd like to explore or make space for. What boundaries do you need to set in order to create space for those *yeses*?

Jack's example: *In order to say "Yes" to <u>more authentically pleasurable sex</u> // I need to start saying "No" to <u>partners who I don't feel comfortable sharing my boundaries with</u>.*

Kira's example: *In order to say "Yes" to <u>a less guilt-ridden, post-divorce sex life</u> // I need to start saying "No" to <u>partners who can't manage their disappointment about my boundaries</u>.*

In order to say "Yes" to _____//
I need to start saying "No" to _____ .

In order to say "Yes" to _____//
I need to start saying "No" to _____ .

In order to say "Yes" to _____//
I need to start saying "No" to _____ .

The High Stakes of Sexually Disappointing Others

How do you look someone in the eye after they've lustfully expressed their desire to cover you in whipped cream and lick it off and respond with a solid, "No way, man. That's just a yeast infection waiting to happen"? How do you tell someone you've been on three dates with, "Sorry, I'm not interested in a fourth" without resorting to ghosting as a way of avoiding the conflict? How do you say no to kissing, a blow job, or a threesome that your partner really, really, *really* wants? How do you tell your new pro-domme that her aim sucks? How do you state a boundary in the moment, during sex, once the ball is already rolling? How do you restate a boundary (yes, again) when a lover just hasn't gotten it quite right (yes . . . *again*)?

How do you sexually disappoint a partner with bravery and confidence? It's become a therapist cliché to quote Brené Brown, but I'm going to do it (again) anyway because, *damn it*, she's right: "Daring to set boundaries is about having the courage to love ourselves, even when we risk disappointing others."[6] There are four key elements to setting solid sexual boundaries neatly packaged in this stellar quote: have courage, love yourself, take risks, and go right ahead and disappoint others.

When we decide not to share our sexual boundaries with our partners out of fear of disappointing them, we are sending the following covert messages:

- Your sexual ego is more important than my sexual pleasure.
- You are not strong enough to survive your own disappointment (and I can't bear to witness that shit).
- Negative emotions have no place in our sexual dynamic (so only share positive ones with me, please).

- I can and want to manage your emotions.
- I don't trust you with my sexual truths.
- I don't want to share my actual sexual self with you.
- I don't feel safe with you.
- I won't tell you my limits, so don't tell me yours.
- You're on your own in figuring out how to have sex with me, and you might step on some sexual land mines while you're at it because I won't be pointing them out to you. Good luck with that.
- I haven't thought about my own sexuality enough to know where my limits lie.
- You are more important than I am.

But when we speak up about our sexual boundaries with any given partner, we set a trend in our sexual dynamic with that partner. When we tell a partner, "No," "Not there," "Never this," "Not quite like that," we are sending the message that:

- My body, emotions, and sexuality are important to me.
- I care about and respect my own boundaries and, therefore, am likely to care about and respect yours.
- Please share your boundaries with me, too.
- I will be an active participant in the sex we have.
- I care about the quality of this sexual interaction.
- I've thought about this.
- I will speak up when something isn't working or didn't work for me so you can relax and feel confident that when things are going right, they're really going right.
- I trust that you can handle my sexual truths and I want you to know them.
- You're not alone in this sexual experience with me, so you

don't need to figure it all out or be in charge of everything.
- I'm here to help guide you in having sex with me—a unique sexual person. You are also are a unique sexual person that I don't dare assume to know everything about.
- My experience of sex matters to me and, therefore, it should matter to you.
- My boundaries matter and so do yours.

When I look at these lists side by side, the benefits of taking the risk to set a boundary far outweigh the possibility of disappointing someone, likely temporarily, and likely (at some point in our long sexual lives) inevitably. The culture of sexual prowess, winning, and accomplishment hurts us all—whether it comes to us in the form of "scoring" sex, being the "most desirable," or being the "best at sex." The problems with this culture of sexual accomplishment are numerous, and among them are these two linked messages:

1. Setting a sexual boundary is perhaps not worth it, lest our sexual partner feel unaccomplished, inadequate, or even just a little hope-dashed (this orients sex as about making your partner feel accomplished rather than connecting to your partner and enjoying yourself), and
2. It's better to be "good at sex" than to be authentically yourself with all of your boundaries, quirks, trauma, desires, and uniqueness (this orients sex as a game that can be won rather than as an organic, customizable experience meant to be enjoyed).

If we were to all build up our internal beliefs in our inherent sexual self-worth and accept our sexual selves as they are, this pattern would eventually undo itself. I would know that setting a boundary doesn't negate my worthiness as a sexual partner, you would know that being told no doesn't negate yours, and we would both be freer to communicate honestly about our shared sex life.

Unfortunately, this is not how most of us have been conditioned to interact with sex. And reconditioning can take some doing. To start small, I would start here: It is okay to feel disappointed. It is okay to disappoint. It is *not* okay to deprioritize the sexual health, safety, and pleasure of yourself or your partner(s) because you have been made to feel responsible for someone else's sexual self-worth.

Let's return to my newly kinky, pro-domme–hiring client, Kira. Kira is in her mid-thirties and freshly out of a long marriage that started too young and took far too long to be ended (by her) after years and years of being left emotionally drained and sexually unsatisfied by her now ex-husband. Thickly padded by their strong friendship and comfortable cohabitation routines, this marriage unraveled slowly and was near-devastating to end for Kira, even though she knew deeply that it was the right choice to do so.

With this marriage came a lot of *shoulds*. Some of them were enforced by family belief systems ("You should not get divorced"), some were handed to Kira via friends ("You're so good together, you should try to work it out"), and many were unspoken and permeated their boring, inorgasmic (for her) sex life. Among these *shoulds* were: "You should be able to orgasm from missionary, penetration-only sex with your husband," "You should not tell your partner that you don't enjoy sex with him," "You should be interested in the same type of sex that your partner is interested in," and "Sex should not be a priority in a long-term relationship."

Kira ended up in my office when all of these messages had rattled around in her brain for so long that she thought she might explode.

Luckily for Kira, she discovered a popular porn site devoted to kinky sex of all kinds. And then . . . finally! Genuine arousal! Curious interest in her own sexuality! Pleasure! Orgasms! Where was Kira to go next, with the *shoulds* of more traditional, vanilla sex in one hand and her porn-playing-phone—I mean her newfound, alternative, and genuine desires—in the other? As with many of my clients, we dove into the work of this book: removing the barriers to discovering and asking for what she authentically wanted out of sex and creating the container (also known as *setting the boundaries*) for that kind of sex life to happen. First, we did a lot of processing of Kira's guilt over not being what her ex-husband had hoped she'd be. Then, we worked to reprioritize her self-worth over her fear of disappointing others. Finally, we explored what she might want to start playing with in her new, kinkier sex life, and Kira got to work setting boundaries that might create the conditions for her genuine desires to thrive.

Kira's Current Boundaries:

- I do not want to date someone who isn't kinky or interested in exploring kink.
- I want to meet potential dates in person first to talk with them about their experience with kinky sex, establish trust, and address any safety concerns.
- I do not want to seriously date anyone right now.
- I want to build friendships with other kinky people via attending local classes and meet-ups.
- I do not want to go out with someone who is only interested in an immediate hook-up situation without getting to know each other first.
- I do not want to start with riskier activities such as rope bondage or impact play. I would rather just utilize fantasy for now.

I Will Know That Someone Is Safe to Explore Kinky Sex with If:

- They have previous experience with kink.
- They have a good knowledge and practice of consent.
- They are friends or acquaintances with other people I know.
- They understand and respect the boundaries I have put in place for our kink play.

Boundaries I'd Like to Reassess at a Future Time:

- If I'd like to explore an emotionally involved, more serious relationship.
- Doing riskier kink activities like rope bondage.
- Being more out about kinkiness to friends and family.

Lastly, Kira did a Yes/No/Maybe List to determine the specifics of what she wanted to, didn't want to, and might want to do with a new kinky sexual partner.

Ultimately, this work helped Kira rewrite her old hurtful messaging that had kept her sexuality and desire underground during her long marriage, and brought her genuine sexuality to the forefront of her post-divorce sex life.

Though permanent damage had been done to her marriage with her husband, Kira was able to reflect on how her fears of disappointing others and their accompanying *shoulds* had kept her silent in her married sex life and had kept her from attempting to share or explore her shifting sexuality with her ex-husband. (Who knows? Maybe if she had been able to bring her interest in kinky sex to her husband, he would've been like, "Oh hey! I'm kinky, too!") Though doing this work to state new boundaries, explore new desires, and take the risk of disappointing others within the context of your relationship can be fruitful in a proactive couples therapy context, doing this work individually can break unhealthy relational cycles that we've been stuck in or are likely to repeat in future relationships.

Meanwhile, in Session with Jack . . .

Jack: I feel like I understand why it's important for me to have this conversation with new partners or at least say something about my desire to avoid blow jobs, but I still don't know how to even have the conversation without coming off like some sort of . . . I dunno . . . unsexy weirdo.

Me: Yeah, I get that—we're definitely lacking in examples and education about how to have these conversations, for sure. Just for fun, let's pretend a friend of yours told you that her Tinder date really wanted to go down on her, she wasn't into it, so she ended the interaction and then the dude said he didn't want to go out with her again. I mean, that's fine, right? No one has to go out with someone again, but do you think you would call your friend "weird," "damaged," or "cunnilingus broken" for having this experience?

Jack: No of course not.

Me: Okay, so then why do this to yourself in almost exactly the same situation?

Jack: I dunno.

Me: If you were the date in that situation—if you were going down on someone and they were having a miserable time, feeling shut down, not into it, and basically panicking— would you want that person to make an excuse and rush out the door? Or would you want them to let you know that they'd like to stop, pause, recalibrate, do something else, or say, "Hey, just to let you know, I don't like people going down on me, can we do XYZ instead?"

Jack: I mean, yeah, probably the second one.

Me: Okay, good. I think I would want that if I were in that situation, too. So, it sounds like you think it's better to set a clear sexual boundary than to suffer in silence, get out of there as soon as possible, and then judge yourself as "broken" later?

Jack: Ugh, yeah.

Me: Okay, cool. I mean, you're definitely not weird for opting for the latter. A lot of people do. But I don't think it's the most solid plan for having the kind of sex you actually want to have.

Jack: Yeah, definitely not. I really don't want this blow job shutdown thing to happen again.

Me: Do you want to make a different plan, then?

Jack: Yeah, let's do it.

How (and When) to Set Your Boundaries with Confidence

You (and your sexual partners) have the power to set the tone in your sexual interactions. If you feel confident and sure about your sexual boundaries, it will be easier to set them. Even if you don't feel super confident, are still learning, or are still exploring your sexual boundaries, you can still confidently tell your partner that this is the case for you. When we set the tone in our sexual interactions, more likely than not our partners will follow suit (if we are attuned to one another), or the opposite will happen, and you will discover a big incompatibility (sooner rather than later, which is usually for the best).

While I always think it's great to have conversations about sexual boundaries before the clothes comes off and we find ourselves vulnerable, turned on, or otherwise in our primal, sexual brains, it's also an excellent idea to have ongoing conversations about your sexual boundaries before, during, and after sex. The following are some examples of how (and when) these sexual boundaries conversations can go.

Before Sex

You, texting: I'm pumped for our date tonight.

Them: Same.

You: Just FYI I had a super long day at work so I'm not sure I'll be down for a long sex session but who knows? Maybe I'll get a second wind.

Them: Okay, cool. I'm actually wicked tired, too, so a make-out and a movie sounds perfect.

You: [emojis]

During Sex

You: OMG you're so fucking hot, I can't even.

Them: *You're* so fucking hot, *I* can't even.

[Starts to go down on you].

You, touching their arm: You know what? I actually get super triggered by people going down on me right off the bat, can we start with hand stuff first?

Them: Oh, sorry, I didn't know that but good to know.

[Still making out, Authentic Mood not dead, I promise.]

Them: Yeah for sure, hand stuff sounds excellent.
[Grabs the lube like a confident loverrrr.]

After Sex

You: Shit, that was great.

Them: It really was.

You: I was really into playing with that bondage rope but I'm realizing that having ties around my ankles makes me feel kind of trapped or something, I'm not sure. But I was really into the wrist restraining.

Them: Oh, really? Seeing you tied up completely with your ankles and your wrists was so hot, but I understand if you're not into it. Do you think if we made the ties looser on your ankles or tried tying you in a different position that you'd feel less trapped and more comfortable?

You: Hmm, I didn't think about that as an option before. That might work! I'm willing to try it out next time as long as we can stop if it gets uncomfortable again.

Them: Yes, of course. Should we make a safe word just so we're super clear about if/when it stops working for you?

You: Yeah, that's a great idea.

Conversations about Sexual Boundaries Can Also Look Like This

Before Sex

You: I want to have sex with you.

Them: I don't.

You: Okay.

During Sex

You: I changed my mind and don't want to do this anymore.

Them: Okay.

After Sex

You: I've done some thinking since we had sex last night and have decided that I'm just not up for a sexual relationship right now.

Them: Okay, did I do something wrong?

You: Nope, not at all. I just want to focus on other things in my life.

Them: Bummer. *[Sad and pouty]*

Them: Are you sure? *[Ego bruised AF; can't seem to get over it]*

You: Yeah, I'm super sure. And also the way you're reacting to this is making me even more sure. This really isn't about you. *[But honestly, now it's starting to be]*

Them, being whiny, so whiny: Okayyyyy, wellllllllllll . . . finnnneee.

You: Okay, well it seems like you're having a hard time hearing what I'm saying right now, and that's fine. But I'm going to go now because I need to meet my sister for lunch.

[Walks away, boundaries and protection of your sexual self so fuckin' intact it's not even funny.]

How to Survive Disappointing Your Lover(s)

To be fearless in setting our boundaries sometimes requires being fearless in disappointing those we love, lust after, like, or simply want to lay. When setting your boundaries, you might know that you are telling a lover something they don't want to hear, which can make setting the boundary feel even more intimidating. However, this doesn't and shouldn't void the necessity of speaking up about what you do and don't want out of sex. After all, if we are to become boundary-setting pros, eventually we will disappoint someone. So, how do you do so with grace and confidence?

Your Lover-Disappointing Survival Guide

First, prepare to disappoint! Think about what experiences or messaging might be contributing to your assumption that your partner will be disappointed by the boundary you are about to set.

Your Turn!
A boundary I'd like to set that I fear will disappoint is . . .

Kira's example: I do not want to date someone who isn't themselves kinky or interested in exploring kink.

Then, check that assumption against what you actually know to be true right now and what the other possibilities might be. What kind of impact do you think this boundary might realistically have on your sexual experience with this person? Will it truly ruin it in the capacity you're thinking it will? Or might it just be a blip that will ultimately enhance your experience because you'll be getting more of what you (both) want and less of what you don't?

Your Turn!

Check your assumptions and beliefs that are contributing to your fear of setting this boundary. Is there any wiggle room to disprove, change, or even just poke a few holes in them? *(What are the other possibilities here of how setting this boundary could go?)*

Kira's example: Kink is becoming more socially acceptable and visible. I live in a liberal area where most people are open-minded. There are probably ways for me to set this boundary via messaging on a dating app instead of face-to-face.

What is contributing to my fear or nervousness about this particular boundary?

(For example: That one time with so-and-so . . . ; I've received

the cultural message from family, friends, and/or media that . . . ; I hold the belief that . . .)

Kira's example: I assume most people are into nonkinky or vanilla sex and therefore will be weirded out by my assertion that an interest in kink is required to date me. I'm nervous that the person wanting to date me will judge me or say something to make me feel embarrassed.

Mentally plan for the best case, worst case, and most-likely case. Best case: you set a boundary, your partner isn't disappointed in the slightest, and you arrive at some shared agreements to make a downright bangin' hook-up happen for you both. Worst case: your partner is a total dick and you don't move forward with being sexual with them at all because they obviously can't handle being told, "No." Most-likely case: your partner is momentarily disappointed by said boundary but you'll be able to chat about what the alternatives are and move on with your sexual day.

Your Turn!
If/when I set this boundary with my partner(s) here's how I think it'll go:

Best case:

Kira's example: I meet someone who is accepting, kinky, and is maybe even kinky in a way that's compatible with my kinkiness!

Worst case:

Kira's example: The person outwardly judges and shames me, setting me back in the work I've been doing to accept and explore this part of myself.

Most-likely case:

Kira's example: In the process of dating, I'll likely meet some people I mesh with and some I don't. This is true whether or not the issue is kink. We could also be incompatible for other reasons. No need to focus on this one particular potential incompatibility. And if for some reason I do feel embarrassed, that feeling will be temporary and will pass.

If my worst-case scenario is realized (which likely it won't be), I would like to react by:

Kira's example: I can end the date and not let the person's judgment or shaming permeate my own beliefs about myself. I could also call a kink-positive friend or talk to my therapist about it to help recover my sense of self from the feelings of being shamed. If someone is that judgmental, they're not a match for me after all.

Next: Set your boundary! As we talked about the above, remember that you can do this as confidently, simply, and calmly as you'd like, and (hopefully, usually) your partner will pick up on the tone you're setting and follow suit. Add some cushion for yourself before you take this risk (whether it feels big or small!).

Your Turn!

If/when I set this boundary with my partner(s), I would like to set the tone! Here are some ways I can think to do that and/or some ways I would like to phrase my boundary: *(Sometimes it helps to practice our phrasing first!)*

Jack's example: Hey, just to let you know, blow jobs are off-limits for me. What's off-limits for you?

Kira's example: For sexual compatibility reasons, I only date other people who are experienced with or curious about kinky sex. If we hit it off and get to that point, do you think we'd be a good fit in this way?

Reminder to myself! I am taking an active part in crafting the most authentic and pleasurable sexual experience for myself and my partner(s) that I can by sharing my boundaries! Here's where I can write some phrases/reminders to hype myself up about why it's important to set this particular boundary and why I'm worth it:

Kira's example: I don't want to repeat the shame and silence around my sexuality that I experienced in my marriage! I deserve to have the sex I truly desire! I've put a lot of work into discovering this part of myself, and pleasing a date is no reason to drop that progress! I'm worthy, worthwhile, and valid, no matter how setting this boundary goes!

Now, let's say your partner is indeed disappointed by this boundary. Disappointed reactions can range anywhere from "Aw, okay" to some sort of passive-aggressive or just outwardly aggressive hissy fit. If your partner chooses this moment to show you that they are not a safe person to disappoint or to set a boundary with, don't have sex with them. If they are a little bummed out by not being able to do certain things with you due to a boundary that you've set, that's okay. They are allowed to have feelings. It's the actions they manifest from these feelings that really count here. Assuming this person is not an unsafe person and you're just dealing with some run-of-the-mill disappointment, here are some things to keep in mind as you proceed:

Remind yourself that setting boundaries is always worth temporarily disappointing others! Remember that you are responsible for your boundaries, your body, and your sexual self. You are also responsible for communicating these with as much clarity (and, if you see fit, kindness) as possible. So good job! You are not responsible for how your partner feels or reacts to these boundaries. Though, if you'd like to, you can take part in helping them work through these feelings (but you are not obligated to). Remind yourself that you're taking an active part in crafting the most authentic and pleasurable sexual experience for yourself and your partner(s) that you can by sharing your boundaries! And, when all else fails, this moment, too, shall pass.

Here are some ways this could go for our friend Jack:

Jack: Hey, before we get sexual, I'd love to hear what you're into or not into, and I'd like to tell you mine, too.
Date: Wow, no one's ever suggested that to me before, but that sounds like a great idea. Should we talk about it now?
Jack: Sure. Shall I start?

Date: Yeah, I need a minute to think about my answers, but maybe if you start it'll help jog my mind.

Jack: Okay, cool. So, I'm super into lots of making out during sex. And dirty talk is great. I'm really not that into getting blow jobs, and I try not to use warming lubes if I can help it because of the gross chemicals.

Date: Hmm, didn't know that about the warming lubes—good to know! I was going to say that I love giving blow jobs, and I do, but I guess that's not in the cards for us. That's okay, though, I'm sure we can figure something else out.

Jack: Yeah, I know it's weird.

Date: No! Not weird at all—I'm glad to know so I don't try to do something you're not into!

Jack: Okay, thanks for being cool about this.

Date: Yeah, for sure, thanks for initiating this conversation, it's super helpful. Let me think more about what some of my *no*s and *yes*es might be . . .

Or maybe . . .

Jack: Hey, before we get sexual, I'd love to hear what you're into or not into, and I'd like to tell you mine, too.

Date: Um . . . okay—that's sort of weird, but I guess we could?

Jack: Oh, I just thought that it would be good to have some general ground rules so we don't accidentally do something that isn't cool with the other person . . .

Date: Yeahhh . . . I guess?

Jack: Do you not want to?

Date: No, it's fine. You start.

Jack: Okay, cool. So, I'm super into lots of making out during sex. And dirty talk is great. I'm really not that into getting blow jobs, and I try not to use warming lubes if I can help it because of the gross chemicals.

Date: Whaattt? What dude doesn't like blow jobs?

Jack, mortified that all of his internalized fears and shame are being proven by this interaction: Um, me?

Date: Yeah, that's weird, I don't know.

Jack, internally reinforced by all of the hard work he's been doing in therapy to undo harmful societal messaging about his unique sexuality and preferences: It's actually really not weird for people to have individual sexual desires and limits, but I'm glad we had this conversation because it's made it clear that we're not really compatible sex partners.

Date: [Explodes into a cloud of sex-shaming dust and disappears forever.]

Disappointment is, of course, not the only reaction we might encounter when we set a boundary for ourselves and a sexual partner. Some of us have experienced less-than-safe responses from past partners or have good, statistical reasons[7] to pay extra attention to the way we let someone down. Though it's great to have these sexual boundary conversations in person when possible, sometimes disappointing someone or outwardly rejecting them can feel safer to do via text, especially if you are LGBTQQIA+ or female-identifying. When in doubt, give yourself permission to communicate your boundaries in whatever way feels safest to you. (For more information about relational violence and safety, head to the resource guide.)

When run-of-the-mill disappointment is our partner's reaction, it may have various origins: your partner may be experiencing the boundary as rejection, or the feedback may be tapping into a fear that they are not good enough, or they may simply be uncomfortable or unfamiliar with the process of talking about boundaries before, during, or after sex. Again, the dominant narrative of sex being something we should be inherently "good at" or should aim to "accomplish" is hurtful to all of us and, we can assume, has also been hurtful to our partners in a variety of ways.

For example, after sex with a new partner, still cuddly in my bed, I asked him what kind of touch had felt good to him and if there was anything he'd like to see happen differently the next time. He stared at the ceiling, mental gears turning, and hands fidgeting in my hair. At first, I took his lack of answers to these gentle inquiries as a pre-rejection; maybe he wasn't interested in building on our sexual experiences together because he didn't see any more in our future. However, after a few more minutes, he revealed that he didn't have answers, not because he was withholding them from me but because he simply did not have them. As a straight, cisgender, white male, he was not used to being asked about the unique aspects of his sexuality or sexual pleasure. He had been raised, like many boys are, under the assumption that he would innately figure sex out for himself, be biologically driven to do so, and, as a man, be inherently easy to please sexually and physically via your basic penile-vaginal sex. By asking about his desires and boundaries, I had simply stumped him. Some people are just not used to being asked about what they like or don't like about sex. In fact, probably many aren't. But don't mistake the newness of this conversation for a lack of necessity. It is likely just the opposite.

How to Have a Sexual Feedback
Conversation (without Being a Dick)

Setting clear sexual boundaries is, at its core, about getting what we want out of sex. And because what we want out of sex tends to change, healthy sexual boundaries can and should have room to evolve. However, many of us struggle to communicate about those evolutions.

Enter the sexual feedback conversation (SFC, for short, or, as it's less gracefully known, *the sexual post-mortem*). There are so many reasons why I love a good SFC:

- It can happen during a time that is not sexually charged, when our heads are clear (and clothes are on), so that we can really articulate what we do/don't want (and maybe even why!).
- Once an SFC has been established as part of the repertoire of a relationship, this can ease the tension of trying to find a way to initiate the conversation, including when and how.
- When used wisely, SFCs can be an intentional time to share new fantasies, ideas, and hopes for your sexual connection, making it more likely that you (and your partner[s]) will get what you want out of sex.
- They make sure your sex life as an individual or with a particular person (no matter how long or short term) is something you're building on and learning from rather than an isolated experience that may or may not be repeated (for better or worse).
- When done tactfully, they can be a bonding, connecting, or trust-building experience for you and your partner(s) and might even be—gasp!—FUN!

Anytime a client reports to me that they don't feel on the same sexual page as their sexual partners, are struggling with an aspect of their sexual experience, or have secret desires that they haven't yet shared (but want to) with their partner, I always ask if they talk regularly about their sex life with their partners outside of sex itself. More times than not, the answer is a sheepish "No," even if it's accompanied by, "but I know it's a good idea." Much like the fear of disappointing others gets in the way of setting proactive sexual boundaries, the fear of hurting our partners' feelings dissuades many from having a good SFC (or any at all).

When I see a couple in my office who is struggling to recreate, renovate, or reinvigorate a slowed or stalled-out sex-life, I make SFCs nearly mandatory.

Brandon and Thom have been together for seven years and have been nearly sexless for three. The couple remembers a sex life fiery and electric in the first two years, routine and regular enough in the third and fourth years, and then less and less present before becoming, in Brandon and Thom's case, almost nonexistent after that. When they scheduled their intake appointment with me, Brandon, self-identified as the higher-desire partner, had gotten sick of wondering if he would ever be able to have sex with his husband again while Thom, self-identified as the uninterested-in-sex partner, was tired of feeling like he was failing or was otherwise completely in charge of the fate of their shared sex life (if only he could rekindle his interest in sex!). Sex had become a touchy topic at home and a silently broiling stalemate had formed in the place where their fiery intimacy used to smolder.

Though we'll hear more about Brandon and Thom and their path toward resolution in Chapter 11, "Navigating Desire Discrepancies," part of the first steps they took during their time in couples therapy was to identify some of the barriers blocking Thom from his genuine desire for sex. Some people don't desire sex and don't want to desire sex, and that's just fine. Other people, like Thom, *want* to feel desire, but no matter how hard they try to muster it up, just can't. For the latter, we start by exploring barriers to desiring.

One of Thom's most powerful barriers, as he discovered, was linked to the origin story of his relationship with Brandon; though Brandon (15 years older than Thom) had been proudly out as gay and sexually exploratory since his early twenties, Thom, now identified as bisexual, had not discovered that he had sexual desires for men until he met Brandon. Though their romantic relationship had flourished and grown into a committed marriage, Thom had given the sexual lead to Brandon as the older, more sexually experienced partner in their sex life.

Though this dynamic had brought a lot of energy into their early sex life, it ultimately left Thom feeling naive, disempowered, and uninterested in his own sex life with Brandon. One of our early pieces of work together was to find new ways to create sexual confidence and to empower Thom through, you guessed it, boundary setting, reinforcing, and adjusting via SFCs. Thom had never really driven the bus of his own sex life and, thanks to the high sex drive and experience that Brandon brought to their relationship, he didn't ever have to. Before Brandon and Thom could rekindle Thom's desire, Thom had to find some kindling to burn: What was *he* into? What kind of sex did Thom want to have (rather than happily having the kind of sex Brandon wanted to have)? How could Brandon and Thom create a safe, boundaried container in which Thom could explore, edit, and home in on these new desires both on his own and in partnered sex with Brandon?

Through a collaborative process that examined each person's role in the sexual cycle between them (more on this in Chapter 11), we began to shift Thom's role toward the research and development arena of their sex life. Meaning Thom began to explore books, erotica, and porn, and reported back to Brandon what he was finding new and interesting about his sexual self and desires via this new sensual media. Then, Brandon and Thom would talk about what pieces of this research they wanted to try implementing in their own sex life and how. Then, after they tried something new in their sex life—things like Thom initiating more often, more eye contact during sex, moving slower, new positions, watching porn together, and so on—they would snuggle in bed with tea and snacks and have a sexual feedback conversation about how the newly introduced sexual experience had gone for each of them, what bore repeating and what didn't, and what they'd like to change for next time.

Throughout this process, Thom explored his desires and also what had been dampening his desire in their pre-therapy sex life. Though shining a light on and then weeding out pieces of their longstanding sexual routine was at times a disappointing process for Brandon, who had thought he was providing Thom with everything he wanted sexually, this process was ultimately an honest bonding experience for both men. And Thom's desire thrived on the newness of their learning experiences together. By introducing SFCs as a mandatory homework assignment as part of couples therapy, Thom and Brandon were able to shed the common illusion that all sexual desire is spontaneous and seamlessly shared equally between long-term partners. Instead, they embraced the idea and the practice that all sexual relationships— especially those that are long-standing—take intentional work, communication, and development.

Like boundaries, feedback has gotten a negative rap, which has stopped too many people from utilizing this important skill in their intimate relationships. Allow me to offer a simple reframe of sexual feedback: It's not about telling your partner that they didn't get it right or are bad at sex. A good SFC is about the two of you collaborating to make the best possible sex life y'all can have, together.

It's true that even when we do our darndest to tell our partners what we do and don't want in bed, they may just not nail it (or us) in the way we were hoping. And it's likely that we may not get something right for them either. And that's okay. We are humans with complex desires, sexual responses, and relationship dynamics. We won't get sex perfectly "right" every time, in every way—no matter how well we know our sexual partners. Rather than looking at sexual feedback like keeping score, grading our partner, or otherwise highlighting all the ways they've failed, a good SFC should capitalize on the teamwork involved in creating good sex.

A good SFC should frame sex as a joint effort and consider that perhaps *we* didn't quite get it right together (instead of *you* didn't get it right). Perhaps something didn't quite click, maybe a directive was misunderstood, or perhaps a new thing y'all tried just didn't work. Rather than let a so-so moment slip by, unacknowledged, in the name of ego or protecting feelings or misplaced guilt, a good SFC seizes said moment as an opportunity for sexual growth, orgasm perfection, or relationship development— together. A good, constructive, useful SFC does not require you to be in a long-term relationship or know your sexual partner that well, and it doesn't require you to hurt their feelings or their egos, or otherwise provide for a negative experience. Simply put: providing sexual feedback doesn't make you a dick, nor does it require you to be one.

Avoid Being a Dick. Don't Make Your SFC about . . .

- Telling your partner they're a sexual failure, "not good at sex," or otherwise "proving" they just don't know you as well as they thought they did.

- Cold-hearted rejection (save that for your sexual rejection conversation, which has its own time and place but should stay out of this one).
- Voiding the enjoyability of the *entire* sexual interaction and all those before it. When SFCs are done consistently, it's clear that they are about editing and adjusting and learning rather than about dropping some big secret bomb that sex has always been silently terrible between the two of you (again, that's another conversation entirely).

Instead, Try Having a Constructive Sexual Feedback Conversation!

- Initiate an SFC during a time you feel connected to and have time to talk to your partner—while you're basking in the afterglow of sex itself, in the car on your day off, or even over text if that's where most of your communicating gets done. Don't throw sexual feedback in the mix of a tense talk, a passive-aggressive tête-à-tête, or an argument about dishes. ("You suck at cleaning up the kitchen just like you suck at giving me an orgasm!!"—not helpful.)
- Package your feedback in a classic compliment sandwich, where constructive criticism is nestled gently between items of positive review: "Wow, that felt so good and my orgasms were intense! I think next time I'd like less dirty talk only because it distracted me from what was happening in my body. But the blindfold was awesome and really heightened the rest of my senses."
- Have an SFC in the spirit of sharing information about yourself and what you like and don't like (e.g., "I don't

like blow jobs," "I see why people like doggy style, but it's not for me," "My clitoris doesn't respond well to super firm pressure") rather than centering around what your partner did or didn't do correctly (e.g., "You suck at blow jobs," "Why do you like doggy style so much? It sucks," "I think you just don't know how to touch clits, dude.").

- Ask your partner to share about their experiences as well. Set the tone for a successful SFC by reacting evenly to the feedback they share with you. Remember that sexual feedback, when shared honesty and kindly, is about your partner telling you about themselves, not about them putting you down or rejecting you as a partner or person.

- Allow yourselves space to discover new things about your sexual responses, desires, and dynamics. Sometimes we are still groping our way toward understanding something and need to talk it out, such as "Something didn't click quite right during that kink scene for me and I don't know why." This can serve as an invitation to your partner to collaborate with you to figure out what didn't sit well, what you might try next time, or where adjustments could be made.

- Have SFCs consistently and often. Though it can be tough to introduce an SFC into a pre-existing sexual relationship, once you get the ball rolling it can be stress-relieving and less negatively charged when it becomes a normal part of your relationship. Also, when you have SFCs regularly, it's more likely that they'll contain both negative and positive feedback, and won't emerge only when things go awry.

- Have SFCs with the goal of working toward the healthiest boundaries for yourself and your sexual partner(s). Remind yourselves (even out loud) that SFCs are a collaborative project toward the mutual goal of your happiest and most pleasurable sex life.

- Resist the cultural messaging that sex needs to be based on competition, accomplishment, and automatic expertise. Because sex is often set up in this way, we are too quick to hear, "You failed," when our partner offers us constructive feedback about a shared sexual experience. Don't let this vibe into your SFC. Instead, lean into communication about your unique sexual selves, about your boundaries (knowing they might change), and sharing about what's real for each of you, including what can be possible moving forward without shame, blame, or sabotaging your sense of self-worth!

In the end, Jack and his blow jobs rode off into the sunset and lived happily ever after. Well, yes and no. As our work together progressed, Jack's therapy goals shifted from wanting to "fix" himself and "just like blow jobs already" to learning more about himself, including how and why messages about masculine sexuality had essentially tricked him into thinking that he needed fixing in the first place. Rather than contorting himself to fit into the idea that "all dudes love blow jobs," Jack learned and practiced new skills in identifying and setting his sexual boundaries with confidence, without (okay, with much less) fear of disappointing his partners, and in a way designed to build his most authentically pleasurable sex life rather than simply check off some blow job based boxes handed to him by cultural assumptions about sex. Did it always go perfectly? Of course not. But, like most of life, good sex doesn't require a lack of work to be done, but instead requires that we learn how to effectively use the tools to do the job. Or, in Jack's case, to not do "the job." (Get it?)

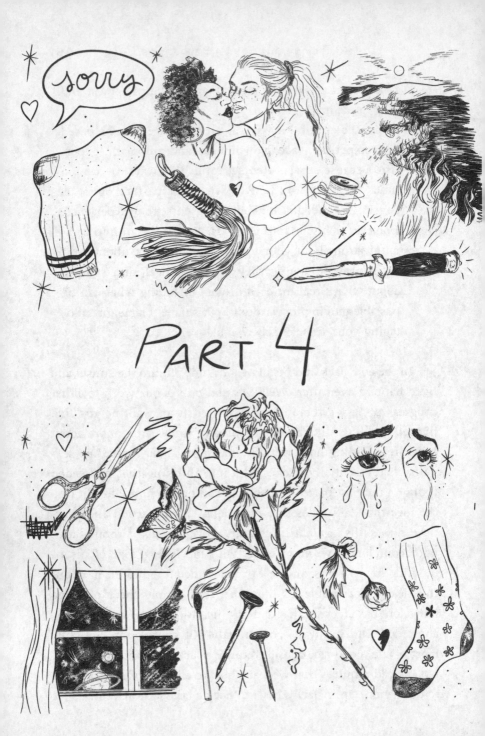

PART 4

Part 4 is all about troubleshooting common sex-life co-nundrums like how to better hear *no* without taking it so personally, what to do if a boundary mistake is made, how to navigate your sex life when you and your partner want different things, and what to do about a libido mis-match. Finally, it will send you on your way with a con-cept called *erotic differentiation*, a relational framework that can guide you through these and almost any other snafu that may come up in your future hot and unboth-ered sex life.

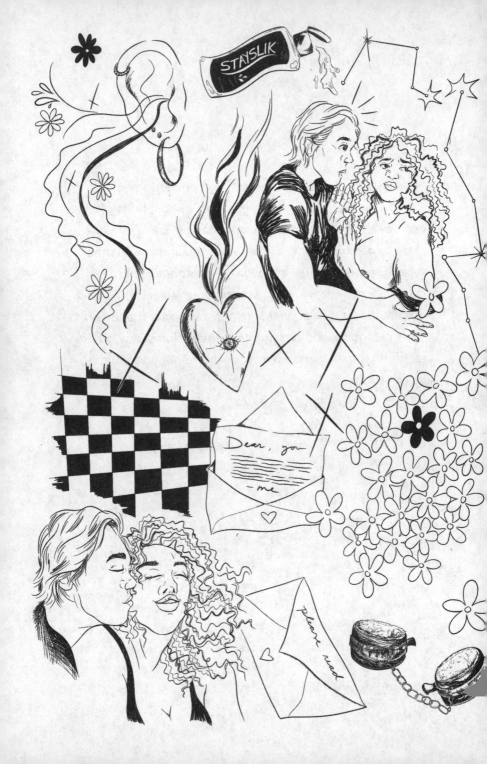

CHAPTER 9

How to Hear *No* Like a Pro

Sometimes *no* is the kindest word.

—*Vironika Wilde, poet and author*

Most of us will take *no* very personally, and we will do so quickly. Even in the healthiest relationships, automatic responses to hearing *no* can include self-doubt, embarrassment, shame, future hesitation at asking for what you want, or emotional shutdown. For many of us, when our partner says *no*, instead of hearing, "This is me sharing my boundaries and desires with you," we are hearing judgments and absolutes like, "I don't want you," "Your desires are shameful," or "You shouldn't have asked me that." These internal reactions are normal, common, and usually happen without much awareness that they are happening at all. They are also unhelpful and counterproductive to consent, authenticity, and genuine pleasure. In fact, how you receive and respond to a partner's boundary is just as important to an authentically pleasurable sex life as learning how to set your own.

No can often sound like a bad word because we are usually taught to equate the word with automatic disconnection and rejection. It's true that sometimes *no* is an outright rebuff or is used to convey a permanent disconnection between you and someone else. It should be obvious by now that you should always respect other people's *no*s, sexual or otherwise. However, this is not always how *no* is used or intended. In the context of what we've been talking about in this book, sometimes *no* and its limit-setting brethren (e.g., "Not like that," "Not right now," and "I'll have to think about that") are actually necessary building blocks to healthy sexual communication. Without the availability and active use of *no*, *yes* loses authenticity, meaning, and enthusiasm. *No* can actually serve as a point of connection—if you let it.

With practice and self-reflection, you can say and hear *no* without disconnection from your partner and, perhaps even more importantly, without disconnection from yourself and your own self-worth. Speaking therapeutically, developing an ease with hearing and responding to *no* starts with building a stronger sense of your individual self in relationship to others. In therapy, we call this lifelong, challenging, transformational process *differentiation*.[1] It is a concept that has informed therapy modalities of all kinds for decades and is crucial in the personal work of hearing and responding productively to your partners' boundaries, limits, hesitations, and *no*s.

In this chapter, we're going to get to know the concept of differentiation well and how it directly applies to our sex lives so that we can comfortably settle into the powerful two-letter word *no* and all of the ways it's a true asset to our best sex lives.

Differentiation 101

Differentiation is a foundational theory of identity development that is utilized by therapists to describe the process of simultaneously defining yourself and your own desires and needs while also remaining connected to your partner(s)', even if your desires conflict with each other. The theory of differentiation posits that if we are able to more clearly delineate our own thoughts, feelings, and beliefs from those of the people closest to us, we will be able to reduce distress in our relationships because we will be more sure of who we are, more accepting of who our partners are, and more comfortable with the differences between the two. If we are well-differentiated, we'll be able to show up in all of our relationships (romantic, platonic, sexual, or otherwise) with more honesty, trust, and closeness *because* we are being more authentic and truer to ourselves, not despite it. At its most basic, differentiation says, "I am me, and you are you, and we can still be us without trying to be one another."

Though there are many, many types of therapy, differentiation is a common thread that runs through nearly all of them. Whether a client is struggling in their marriage, with a family member, having anxiety about work and friendships, or feeling depressed about their life circumstances, nudging a client toward differentiation is a common and helpful path through the emotional muck. Practicing differentiation is helpful in nearly every single scenario. When we're living a well-differentiated life, we're better able to feel secure and sure of our own worth, values, and sense of self. We're less likely to over-compromise, shrink, or sabotage our own boundaries in relationships with other people. We're also less likely to feel the need to control the thoughts, actions, and beliefs of those around us, which also greatly diminishes relationship killers like resentment, bitterness, and stalemates.

Differentiation makes many appearances in the sex therapy I do with clients. Though most romantic and sexual relationships are built on the lore that agreeing, being similar, and having zero conflict makes for the healthiest and strongest connections, differentiation begs to differ. Instead, differentiation looks at how our differences are inevitable, how conflicting desires can push us to grow in our relationships, and how we can resist compromising ourselves for what we *imagine* is best for our relationships (spoiler alert: compromising yourself is rarely best for the relationship). This comes in handy when tackling common sex therapy topics such as desire discrepancies, sexual self-discovery, improving boundary setting and communication, and reducing sexual shame and self-judgment (we'll get more into this soon).

The concept of differentiation is not new and it's certainly not mine. Differentiation was originally developed by family therapy heavy-hitter Murray Bowen in the 1950s.[2] It also hugely informs the modern-day Developmental Model of Couples Therapy[3] created by Ellyn Bader and Peter Pearson,[4] which I am grateful to have heavily studied early on in my therapy career. Differentiation is essentially the cornerstone of relational therapy of all kinds, so there are a lot of—typically heavily academic and heady—ways to talk about what it means. Which is to say, forgive me, psychotherapy elders, for the simplifications I'm about to make here, starting with baseball and ending with Venn diagrams.

Not Another Baseball/Sex Analogy

Imagine: You've just had a stellar first date with a new person—they're charming, funny, polite to your waiter, have the most captivating eyes you ever did see, and the dinner conversation flowed like sweet, sweet honey. They text you a couple of days later inviting you to a baseball game. They *love* baseball. Not only do they find baseball games to be fun and relaxing (in that rowdy, energetic kind of way) but it also makes them nostalgic for their childhood when their dad used to coach their Little

League games (how adorable!). Though baseball has never really been your thing, you (of course!) say yes because going to this game certainly won't be torture, and it sounds like a cute date idea. During the game your date is really in their element. The peanuts are popping, the chants are contagious, and by the end of the sixth inning, you find yourself in swoon city. It's a regular ol' falling-in-love movie montage over here. "Dang," you think, "this person could stick around for a *while*."

Turns out, they do. Six years later you've got a kid, a house, and season tickets to these fucking baseball games. The bleachers are uncomfortable, the concession food gives you heartburn, and all the yelling gives you a headache. But baseball games have become your relationship's *thing*. Beyond being a seasonal tradition, it's played a leading role in your how-we-met story and has created an important place for your partner to connect their past to their present life with you. It's not just baseball; it's emotional, relational, and has become a strong tether between the two of you, especially for your partner.

Personally, your patience for baseball ran out a long time ago. Though early in your relationship you happily bent the rules of your own interests in favor of nurturing all the ways you could connect to this new person, here in your established partnership of the present, you'd rather spend the time and energy of these baseball games on your own interests and other relationships with friends, family, and your child. In fact, you're starting to become downright resentful of all this time and money that you're spending on your partner's baseball fanaticism rather than on your own life. When's the last time they spent the equivalent of six years of baseball season tickets on *you* and *your* interests?

You want to bring up the idea of significantly cutting back on your baseball attendance or, really in an ideal world, you'd like to stop going altogether, but you're worried about what this might mean to your partner, how they might feel about it, and what this shift could do to your relationship. The truth is that you've never liked baseball and that at the start of your relationship with this person, you downright exaggerated your interest in it because it felt good to connect and you wanted them to like you. To admit this now might cause strife, a feeling of betrayal, or at the very least rock your otherwise smooth(ish)-sailing boat. The unknown repercussions and fear of disconnect from your partner encourage you to stay quiet, and you keep going to baseball games in the name of maintaining the status quo of your relational connection, all the while obscuring your partner's ability to see you thrive in the other areas of *your* life you've been neglecting—all in favor of *their* (not your) love of the game.

Can you relate to this or a similar scenario in a past or present relationship? How might this play out for each person in this story if instead of baseball we were talking about the established desires and routines in their sex life? Where in your sex life or relationships have you hemmed in the edges of your boundaries and desires in order to satisfy the other person or to maintain the current security of your connection? How have you done this or are you doing this in your relationships in the name of reducing (real or imagined) conflict, tension, or hiccups to your relational harmony? Is doing this actually creating connected compatibility? Or just the illusion of it? This is a lack of differentiation at work. But lack of differentiation is also normal and common because, ultimately, it comes from the deep desire to maintain connection,

stability, acceptance, and love. If you see yourself or your relationship in this little baseball story, you're not alone, you're just
human. And, just like my clients, you're capable of differentiating
for the better.

Though I've never actually had clients come in with baseball-
themed complaints, I have fielded many other 75-minute-long
couples therapy sessions about similar, seemingly trite issues: She
never hangs up her wet towels; the way he chews his cereal is
sickening; he does all of the dishes save for five utensils he just
leaves there in the sink! Of course, these issues are never *actually* about towels and cereal. They're stand-in examples for larger
cycles of relational strife with deeper meaning. She doesn't pay
attention to detail (or to me), he's inconsiderate (I don't matter),
or maybe we're just not compatible (what does it mean for our
relational longevity if we can't even agree on the way dishes are
done?). Though the couples in my office often look at me sheep-
ishly or flat-out apologize for bringing in such "boring topics,"
the truth is that these types of issues are common, and they are
important. These conversations illustrate our experience of our
relationship, our perception of our partner, and our level of sure-
ness in ourselves; they can also tell us a lot about where we're at
in our own process of differentiation.

According to Bader and Pearson's Developmental Model of
Couples Therapy,[5] it's incredibly normal for all relationships to
have a certain "status quo" or collection of unspoken rules that
each partner (usually subconsciously) strives to maintain. It may
look like the above example of baseball season tickets or it might
show up in cycles like the division of domestic labor, who storms
off in a fight and who shuts down, or who initiates sex and how
the sexual interaction tends to go after that. According to Bader
and Pearson's therapy model, it's also to be expected that at some

point one, both, or all of the people in a relationship will begin to shift away from prioritizing the status quo and toward (re)prioritizing their own individual interests, boundaries, or other previously obscured truths about themselves. This is a predictable pattern that all relationships move through that Bader and Pearson have laid out in four distinct relationship stages[6]:

1. Symbiosis: That can't-get-enough-of-you, no-couple-has-what-we-have honeymoon phase. Polyamorous circles call this *new relationship energy*.[7] I call it being high on oxytocin,[8] also known as *the bonding hormone* that's released during physical intimacy. However you label this fresh relationship phase, you know it when you see it (or feel it) and, sadly, it's always temporary. This is also the shortest relationship phase; some relationships continue on after it's done, and some don't.

2. Differentiation: The driving force in this chapter and the second relational stage, where each person in the relationship starts to notice more acutely what's different about each of them and often struggles heartily (and usually subconsciously) to either accept, assimilate, or otherwise erase those differences. This is a stage that can last years and that some couples make it through and some don't. This is also the stage during which most couples start couples therapy.

3. Exploration: The stage where each person in the relationship begins to really explore themselves and what they want, individually. This phase can feel scary, threatening, and destabilizing as many people in relationships erroneously equate independent thoughts, feelings, desires, and pursuits as an indicator of inevitable separation or a

threat to their connection. In fact, it's quite healthy to be a fully formed, individual person with your own thoughts, feelings, and beliefs, even when you're in a relationship with another person. It's also quite healthy to be different from your partner (you are not the same person, after all).

4. Rapprochement: The holy grail of Bader and Pearson's model of relationships. This is when we've made it over the rainbow and over our fears of our differences. In this phase we are able to embrace ourselves as separate individuals and see our relationship as a thriving force not in spite of our differences but because of them. The word Bader and Pearson use often to describe this phase is *vitality*.[9]

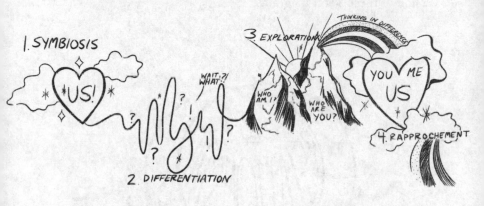

When a new couple starts therapy, they've usually just hit the differentiation fork in the road and relational tensions have risen to the surface as a result. Usually one person has begun the process of differentiating ("I don't want to spend my time at baseball games anymore," "I think I'm non-monogamous," "Wait, my orgasm issues aren't about something being wrong with me; I'm just having the wrong kinds of sex for me!") and the other person is either scrambling to catch up or, more likely, reaching out to pull the other person back into comfortable symbiosis ("But you buy us season tickets for my birthday every year!", "What if I just give you a 'free pass' to sleep around once a year?", or "Does this mean you've never enjoyed the sex we have this entire time?"). Sometimes, a couple has taken the opposite, avoidant route through differentiation, skirting their differences entirely by building a chasm of distance, coolness, and detachment between them (usually this type of couple doesn't bother to come to couples therapy). When either of these types of couples come in and describe these kind of presenting problems to me, I introduce the concept of differentiation to them by talking about baseball (a sport I truly know nothing about) and then drawing my quick version of these Venn diagrams:

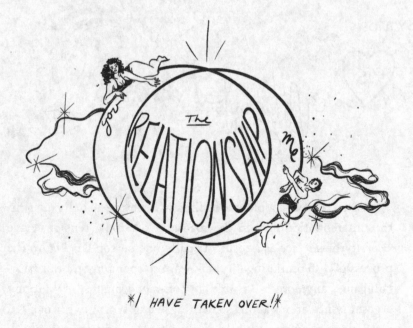

Figure 1

Figure 1 depicts being enmeshed at the beginning of a relationship. The *we* has taken over, and the *I* and the *you* have become almost unrecognizable. This couple will say things like, "*We* have a hard time communicating and *we* could *both* use some anger management help" rather than saying, "*I'm* prone to lashing out during arguments and *I'd* like to stop doing that because *I* can see that it hurts my partner and our relationship." This is the type of relationship that, when it ends, one or both people will come out of unsure of who they are on their own or may pleasantly exclaim, "Wow! I forgot how much I love painting!" or some other previously cherished hobby that they completely dropped during the relationship.

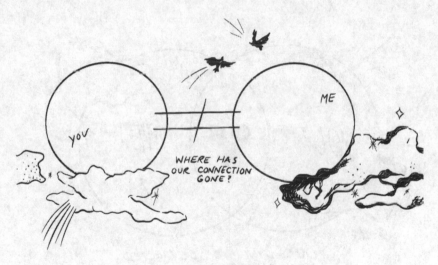

Figure 2

Figure 2 depicts an overly individuated pair of people who, by default, believe that they are in a relationship though in reality they do very little relating. This couple usually sits on the couch in my office and, upon learning about differentiation, proudly exclaims,

"Oh! We're really good at that—we rarely ever spend any time together. We're *very* independent." The individuals in this relationship are on the opposite end of the spectrum from enmeshment, not
because they thrive in their differences, but because they fear that
without maintaining a certain distance between them, the things
that are important to them as individuals may collapse into over-
compromising all too easily. Just like the enmeshed couple in Figure
1, their boundaries and sense of self aren't strong enough to withstand differentiation, they just manage it in the opposite way. As
a result, they operate side by side in disconnection, making for a
relationship that may fizzle out on its own, without much fanfare,
or may just continue in unsatisfactory stagnation for ages.

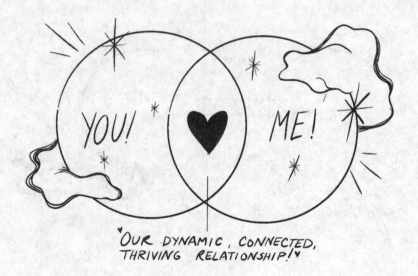

OUR DYNAMIC, CONNECTED, THRIVING RELATIONSHIP!

Figure 3

Figure 3 is what we're shooting for.[10] This Venn diagram depicts two individuals who are well-defined and recognizable to

themselves, as themselves. They know who they are, how they're different from their partner, and what keeps them connected together. They each work equally to nourish their own interests *and* their relationship. Between them, their relationship takes up a Goldilocks amount of space, time, energy, compromise, conflict, agreement, and disagreement—not too much, not too little, just the right amount. This well-differentiated relational state also happens to be very good for your sex life.

Erotic Differentiation

The opportunity to practice differentiation in your sex life will arise in nearly every element of an authentically pleasurable sex life: discovering what you want, sharing your desires with your partner(s), asking for what you want, asking your partner(s) what they want, setting your own boundaries, and receiving your partner(s)' boundaries with grace and acceptance. What I call *erotic differentiation* is essentially created by defining your sexual self clearly and bravely while allowing your partner(s) to freely do the same— yes, especially when those sexual selves don't perfectly align. (Remember, differentiation is all about thriving *because* of inevitable difference, not in spite of it or by squashing it). Though differentiation is a multilayered, complex psychotherapy theory, the small, attainable things you can do to push yourself toward becoming well-differentiated in your sex life are actually quite ordinary, yet very impactful.

Partners who are struggling with erotic differentiation may present as either enmeshed (as illustrated in Figure 1) or overly individuated (as illustrated in Figure 2). Some partners may even toggle between the two as they wrestle with developing a sexual relationship that can withstand and even welcome difference.

Though every sexual relationship is unique to the people in that sexual relationship, there are some common, concrete ways that erotic differentiation can manifest in an otherwise safe and healthy relationship.

A Person Struggling with or Avoiding Erotic Differentiation Might:

- Be able to identify a specific sexual desire they have but will wait for their partner to bring it up first. This person is also willing to never explore this desire if their partner never brings it up.
- Fake an orgasm in order to avoid the conflict that may arise from being honest with their partner about their lack of climax.
- Fold their boundaries quickly and easily, especially if they perceive that doing so will please their partner.
- Globalize any "Not right now," "No," or similar boundary from their partner as a complete and everlasting rejection.
- Struggle to answer sexually self-defining questions such as "What do you want?" or "How do you like to be touched?" even when they know the answer.
- Assume a lack of sexual frequency in the relationship indicates a problem in the relationship itself without talking to their partner about it (of course, sometimes it does but not always).
- Consider their in-the-moment sexual needs (such as wanting more lube, to shift positions, or to take a pee break) as a nuisance that's not worth bringing up.
- Avoid (consciously or subconsciously) asking their partner relevant questions about their sexual self or for feedback about their present-day shared sex life.

- Pretend that neither partner engages in a personal sex life such as masturbation, porn consumption, or fantasizing, even if it's an open secret that they most definitely do. These partners may never ask to incorporate these elements into partnered sex even though they would enjoy it or want to.
- Feel easily replaced by a sex toy or wouldn't bring up their desire to incorporate toys so as not to offend their partner.
- Quickly drop their personal interest in a new desire, kink, sex position, sex toy, or other sexual experience if they receive any kind of disagreement, judgment, or anything less than an automatic shared personal interest. For example, this person might broach the topic of wanting to be blindfolded during sex and if their partner's response is, "Oh really? Why do you want to be blindfolded?" they might take this question as a reason to shut down, brush off, or otherwise halt further conversation entirely.
- Consciously or subconsciously shift their sexual interests to match their partner's. For example, if Partner A is really into kinky sex but Partner B likes both kinky and vanilla sex equally, Partner B might find themselves watching more kink-focused porn than vanilla-focused porn, or neglecting their desire for vanilla sex to be incorporated into their shared sex life.
- "Go with the flow" of sex to the detriment of their own wants and boundaries, such as allowing the other person to set the pacing of sex, the content of sex, or the timing of sex in a way that, even though consensual, prioritizes their partner's desires, feelings, or interests above their own.
- Struggle to set clear boundaries, especially if their clear boundary is to say *no* to something their partner really, really, really, really desires.

- Fail to bring up something that isn't going well overall or that they didn't like in a recent shared sexual experience with their partner. Instead, they bury it, ghost the other person over it, or wait for the other person to (hopefully) bring it up or figure it out on their own.

- Cut themselves off from sex entirely (different than simply being asexual[11] or not interested in sex) because they don't trust that they will be able to interact with a sexual partner in a way that balances each partner's sexual desires, boundaries, wants, and needs while simultaneously practicing healthy self-advocacy (different than asserting pressure or making demands).

Conversely, Partners Who Are Actively Moving toward Erotic Differentiation:

- Assume and acknowledge that each person in the relationship has a unique sexual history that has helped shape the sexual person they are today.

- Are able to have open and honest conversations about their sexual wants and needs, even when those wants and needs do not seamlessly overlap (see Chapter 11).

- Ask curious, open-ended questions of their partners when they bring up a new sexual interest that they themselves either haven't heard of, feel some judgment or shame about, or feel threatened by.

- Engage in critical self-reflection about their own thoughts, feelings, and reactions to their partner's desires, boundaries, and limits.

- View their personal sexuality as an ongoing discovery about themselves and take ownership over regularly checking in with their current boundaries, limits, and desires.

- Confidently assert their sexual boundaries even when a relationship is new or if that boundary will drastically shift the dynamic of a longer-term relationship.
- Say *no* with clarity and care for the other person.
- Are able to advocate for their own sexual needs and desires during a sexual interaction, even as the interaction is currently unfolding.
- Come back around to a sexual interaction or discussion as new information becomes available, such as realizing their feelings have changed about a sexual interaction or desire (e.g., "I thought I was okay with it, but now something feels unsettling," "I realized why I like this certain kink so much," "Actually, XYZ desire *is* really important to me, even though I let it go really easily in our last conversation").
- Can identify their sexual needs, wants, boundaries, and limits within themselves as well as the appropriate time to share them with their sexual partner.
- Explore their own changing, inner sexual world on an ongoing basis, and can determine who to share this inner world with and how, or is at least willing to practice that part.
- Honor their own level of desire for sex (sex drive) without value judgment around being the higher- or lower-desire partner. Consider this difference to be common and likely in longer-term relationships.
- Define the success of their sex life based on whether or not it's working for the people within that sex life and not based on the frequency per week or "spicing-things-up-ness" of other people around them.
- Consider their partner as their own unique sexual being with their own thoughts, feelings, desires, boundaries, sexuality, gender, and sexual experience and history.

They don't assume to know the totality of this unique sexual being and don't expect to.

- Respect their partner's sexual privacy and don't feel entitled to know all sexual thoughts, feelings, and experiences that their partner has (of course, all agreed-upon relationship boundaries are assumed respected here). Instead, these partners invite each other to share things about their sexual selves with curious questions and nonjudgmental reception.

- Utilize creativity and externalized problem-solving when their desires don't match up (way more on this in Chapter 11).

Basically, active erotic differentiation looks like Figure 6 rather than Figures 4 or 5.

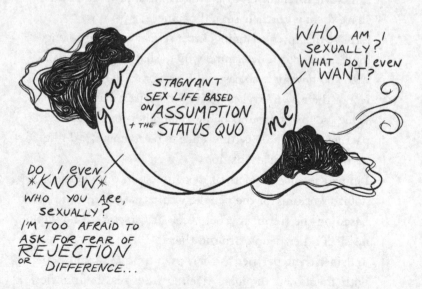

Figure 4

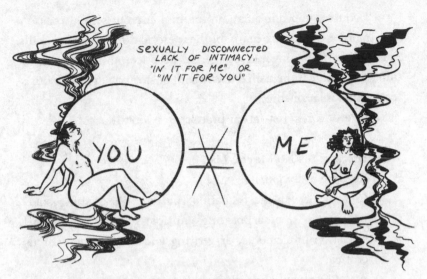

Figure 5

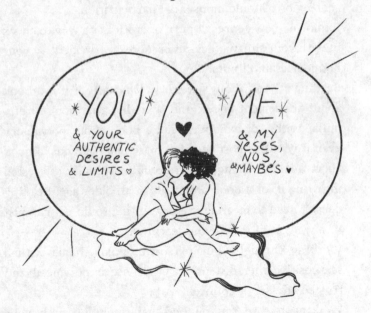

Figure 6

Of course, you don't have to be in a current sexual relationship in order to practice many of these erotic differentiation skills. Most of the following personal, solo practices to increase erotic differentiation can be utilized whether or not you are in a consistent sexual relationship.

Solo erotic differentiation practice can look like:

- Doing a Yes/No/Maybe List!
- Keeping a sex journal.
- Creating lavish masturbation routines like making solo home videos, incorporating multiple sex toys or kinky sensation implements, or writing and reading your own erotica.
- Attending sexuality classes that involve group thought sharing or platonic, nonsexual participation.
- Exploring new genres of porn or erotica as a way to check in with your shifting desires or more clearly identify your boundaries and limits.
- Reading a book about sexuality, especially if it is a book about an element of sex and sexuality that you're unfamiliar with. For example, read a book about polyamory even if you're almost certain you're monogamous, a book about anal sex though you're only marginally interested in trying it, or a book about sex at an older age. Reading doesn't need to mean doing or wanting to do—it can just be a way of informing and learning.
- Working through your personal sexual shame with a sex-positive therapist or an otherwise experienced and trusted adviser or counsel.
- Working toward finding personal resolution with your own desires and sexuality, even if it stands in contrast to

the social messages you've received about your sexuality or if/when they are different than those of your peers or past partners (e.g., being queer in a conservative area, having an interest in kink when everyone you know is purely vanilla, enjoying anal sex as a straight cisgender man).

A lack of erotic differentiation can include a series of small actions that can add up quickly to make sex about performance (making assumptions about the other and "pleasing" them based on those assumptions) rather than about authentic pleasure (actively inquiring and talking about each person's desires and co-creating a mutually pleasing experience). On the other hand, actively working toward erotic differentiation includes both getting to know your sexual self honestly and clearly while also making ample, welcoming space to get to know your partner's sexual self, even when this process risks finding out that your sexual selves might not perfectly align.

In Bader and Pearson's Developmental Model of Couples Therapy, the big push toward differentiation happens right after the la-la-land, we'll-always-want-the-same-things-and-never-struggle symbiotic stage. There are many ways that differentiation can come and smack you with the reality that you and your partner are different people who might actually not always be perfectly compatible (Normal! Fine! Healthy even!). There are two common ways that the symbiotic stage is challenged and the differentiation stage is introduced in an otherwise healthy, communicative, and consensual sexual relationship, specifically: 1) when partners reach a seemingly impossible-to-navigate difference in desire (also known as *desire discrepancy*, covered in Chapter 11), and 2) hearing *no* or a similar boundary from our sexual partner, which we'll explore here with Sam and Nadine.

Sam and Nadine: Hearing No Is Hard to Do

When I teach my workshop "Consent and Cookies"[12] at high schools, I teach practical, age-appropriate consent strategies for youth that they can utilize in their current dating lives and in their future, adult sex lives. At the end of the workshop, we put these new consent skills into practice with a fun, cookie-decorating and communication activity. Somewhere in the lecture portion, we cover the value of hearing *no* like a pro. To do this, I say to the group of teens, "You just went out on a first date. At the end of the date, the person asks you if they can kiss you. You say, 'Not tonight, I'd rather wait.' Now, who would you rather go on a second date with? The person who hears you say *no* to their kiss request by saying, 'No problem, I hope you have a good night and I look forward to a second date if you'd like one'? Or the person who does this?" and then I pretend to throw a big ol' pouty fit about not getting my way. When I ask the group to raise their hands if they want a second date with Person 1 or Person 2, it's a clear sweep in favor of Person 1 save for the occasional class clown who wants to advocate for the fit-thrower. Of course, this isn't the only bit of education we do about why it's important to listen to and respond to a *no* with respect, kindness, and even gratitude, but it makes its point— hearing *no* with grace makes your dating experience better for everyone involved, including you.

I also make this point with my adult clients in couples therapy but usually it takes longer, with a little more finesse and fewer dramatics on my end. For example, Nadine and Sam, a couple in their early 60s, have been together for many years and have had a largely successful, long-standing sex life throughout their relationship. However, following her recent retirement, Nadine's sense of purpose and sense of self began to slip away, including her normally high desire for sex. As is the case with most people, Nadine's insight about the connection between the end of her working years and her nose-diving sex drive didn't occur to her until many months later, and certainly wasn't made apparent to Sam until we were well into therapy. During the year prior to starting therapy, this classic miscommunication created an unhelpful cycle in Nadine and Sam's relationship: the more Nadine turned Sam's sexual advances down due to her own depression, low self-worth, and subsequent lack of interest in sex, the more frustrated Sam got—not just because she wanted to have fun and satisfying sex with Nadine like they always had, but because she was experiencing the kind of frustration with roots more deeply embedded in her own fears of inadequacy, aging, and unlovability coupled with the despondency that accompanies countless unspoken and unanswered questions.

By the time Nadine and Sam found themselves in couples therapy with me, sex had come to a complete halt and Nadine had started avoiding Sam's touch and even conversations about sex all together. Sam, on the other hand, had doubled-down on her efforts to "solve the problem" including suggestions of books, classes, and even medical avenues that she thought Nadine could and should explore to "get her sexuality back." In the typical push-pull dynamic that can crop up in such a relational dynamic where one person pursues the other while the other person retreats further away the more the first one pursues, Sam's efforts to "help" had become a big hindrance, made even bigger by the fact that underneath Sam's "helping" motivation lay a subconscious goal to prove herself adequate, lovable, and wanted.

The tighter this cycle of push-pull wound around Nadine and Sam, the higher the stakes of rejection climbed. And this is when they decided couples therapy was in order. After a few months, we reached a point in our work together where Nadine and Sam had shared their inner stories and reflections about what had happened in their sex life to cause its drastic decline, and Nadine in particular was feeling more ready than ever to pick up their sex life again. However, there was now a newer barrier for her to navigate before she could jump in the sack with confidence once more: though Nadine was feeling far more interested in sex with Sam again, Sam continued to respond to Nadine's boundaries, feedback, preferences, or anything else she may perceive as yet another rejection in unhelpful ways. Understandably, the past year of repeated and seemingly sudden (to Sam) rebuffs, rejections, *no*s, and *not now*s from Nadine had really stacked up on Sam's end. Without having asked Nadine about her experience, and without Nadine having shared the connection between her loss of personal purpose and her loss of desire for sex, Sam had spent the year before they entered therapy making some assumptions of her own in an attempt to connect the dots and solve their problem. In reality, Nadine's initial lack of desire was more about herself than about Sam. However, the overly personal way Sam received Nadine's *no*s had snowballed over time into another layer of dysfunction preventing their sexual connection, a layer we began to lift in our second half of therapy together.

"I worry now that any time I say, 'No' or 'Not like that' or 'Let's try later' or even 'Can you shift a little to the right?' that Sam is just going to get that look on her face—yeah! That one!" Nadine says, pointing at Sam's dejected facial expression, happening in real time during one of our sessions.

Sam lightheartedly rolls her eyes and says, "What?! It's hard to be rejected for over a year and not know why, okay?"

"You're both right," I tell this couple before they can head off to the races of defending their individual points. "It's not sexy to have someone pout when you're trying to tell them what you want in bed, and it's not fun feeling repeatedly rejected. So, what are we going to do about this if the two of you want to have sex together?" I ask this last question to help reorient them back to their shared goal: to get their sex life back on track.

"Well," Nadine says, "Sam can stop pouting, for one."

"That would probably help, yes," I agree. "But first, before you make an ask of Sam, I'm more interested in what you're going to do, Nadine, for yourself, rather than what Sam is going to do for you. Remember, you're going to feel more capable of change if the change is up to you, not up to Sam."

This is something my long-standing clients are used to: I ask them to talk about their own missteps, change points, and actions rather than their partner's. This is one way to practice differentiation in therapy. I often do this with clients by interrupting a story they're telling about all of the things their partner did wrong in this week's argument with the question, "What's something *you* did in this argument that made things worse?" Not only does this kind of self-orientation help clients practice accountability but it is also a small and impactful way to practice differentiation, especially when this refocusing is repeated over time.

It's easy to point at the other person and say, "They did this" and "They always do that" but it's harder (and more important) to look toward oneself and say, "I'm untrue to my values when I _____," "I contribute unhelpfully to this situation when I _____," "I can change this cycle positively if I'm willing to _____." When we shift away from pointing at the other and turn inward to the self in this way, we are practicing differentiation because we are getting in touch with our own values, boundaries, and behaviors rather than making it our mission to force our partner to have the same values, boundaries, and behaviors that we do.

Rather than attempting to get the other person back in line (or back to symbiosis), we can practice differentiation by considering what we can do to better manage differences between ourselves and our partners instead of wasting our energy attempting to obliterate those uncomfortable differences entirely. When we resist trying to force the other person to change, we acknowledge that our partner also has a personal set of values, boundaries, and limits that are just as important as our own. Rather than ignore or stamp our differences out, a person moving toward differentiation will take control of their own parts of the unhelpful relationship cycle at hand, starting with the question, "What did I do to make this worse and what can I do to make it better?"

In answering this question for herself, Nadine decided that she could help Sam not take her boundaries so personally by following them up with an alternative option for connection. For example, instead of saying, "I don't want to have sex tonight" and walking away to do something else (initiating disconnection), she wants to try saying, "I don't want to have sex tonight but I would love to cuddle and watch a movie" (maintaining connection).

"That sounds like a great option," I tell Nadine. "Sam, do you think that would be a helpful shift for you?" Sam says it would and that it would help remind her that just because Nadine doesn't want to have sex doesn't mean that she doesn't want *her*.

Then, it's Sam's turn. Sam talks to Nadine and me about the ways she thinks her current reactions to Nadine's rejections (no matter how large or small) are probably not stoking Nadine's sexual fires (to no surprise, Nadine agrees).

"So, what do you think you need to do in order to shift your reactions in a helpful way?" I ask.

"Well, I just take it so personally," she says. "It feels like it's just another brick on my back when I'm already carrying so many after this last year of constant barriers between us."

"Sounds like you need to unload some of those bricks," I suggest.

Sam agrees, and this is where some of her own erotic differentiation homework begins.

How to Treat No Like It's Good for Your Sex Life (Because It Is)

When, like Sam, you set out to get better at hearing *no*, start with an inventory of your triggers and reactions, followed by some positive motivation to help keep you on track. Below is a worksheet that encapsulates some of the conversations I have with clients when we are working on this task, distilled into questions and prompts for you to do at home. Of course, this work can be done on a deeper level with a therapeutic professional. This worksheet aims to get you to dig a little deeper into yourself and to get curious about your own particular brand of reactivity to rejection.

Reflections on My Reactions to "No"

Hearing *no* is hard. It can bring up challenging feelings, poke old childhood wounds, or seem to confirm a deeply held fear about our self-worth or lovability. If we want to feel stronger in the face of *no*, and therefore more capable of responding to it with grace and acceptance, we first need to understand why it's so challenging in the first place.

There are three different sections of self-reflection about what happens for you internally (feelings and emotional responses) and externally (behaviors and actions) when you hear *no* or a similar boundary: 1) self-evaluation 2) relational ripple effects, and 3) sweet reminders to keep you moving toward the goal of hearing *no* like a pro. Remember, this is a starting point, not a cure-all, so go easy on yourself and note the areas that could use more in-depth work outside of what this book and worksheet can provide.

Self-Evaluation

How Do I Feel? What Do I Do? Where Does This Get Me?

When I Hear *No* or a Similar Boundary, I Feel:

(Circle all that apply or add some of your own.)

Angry	Rejected	Hurt	Lonely
Like I did something wrong	Like I'm being punished	Childish	Embarrassed
Ugly	Undesirable	Uncomfortable	Accused
Confused	Sad	Disappointed	Ashamed
Shamed	Numb	Curious	Grateful
Relieved			

Other:

When I Hear *No* or an Undesired Boundary, I:

(Circle all that apply or add some of your own.)

Shut down	Retreat	Get quiet	Push my partner away
End the interaction	Backpedal (i.e., try to water down or take back what you had asked for or said)	Sulk	Reject my partner
Defend myself	Cry	Avoid that boundary in the future	Try to remain open
Remind myself of my self-worth	Note what I've learned about my partner		

Other:

When I respond poorly to a boundary, I hope that my partner will respond by:

However, I make it harder for them to respond this way because:

I learned to respond to boundaries in unhelpful ways from:

(Hint: Does this behavior ring true in other or past areas of your life or people you have learned from?)

It is my responsibility to change these unhelpful patterns. It's beneficial to me and my relationships if I change these unhelpful patterns because:

Relational Ripple Effects

How Does Hearing *No* Like a Pro Help My Relationship?

Some other more productive responses to *no*/boundaries that I would like to try are:

____ Thanking my partner for telling me

____ Taking a deep breath before I respond

____ Reminding myself not to take a boundary personally

____ Giving my partner space to make decisions

____ Repeating back to my partner what I've heard so they know I understand

____ Staying emotionally open to my partner rather than closing off to protect myself

____ Asking my partner what they'd like to do instead of simply saying, "Okay!" without pouting

____ Sitting with or writing about my own disappointment or triggers later on my own/with a friend

Other:

I think these new responses will help me maintain connection because:

If/when I'm able to respond more productively to my partner's boundaries, I imagine that this will allow them to feel:

Sweet Reminders

Soothing Self-Talk and Positive Reframes to Use When Hearing *No*

When I welcome *no* or a boundary, I also welcome _____
_____ into my sex life.

When my partner is sharing a boundary, they are telling
me: _____
_____.

They are not telling me: _____
_____.

Something I love and appreciate about my partner's
boundaries:

Something I love and appreciate about myself:

Beyond doing her own personal insight work about the roots
and triggers of her automatic reactions to boundaries, there are sev-

eral concrete skills that Sam has learned in couples therapy that have contributed to her increased erotic differentiation. These include learning and practicing more productive ways to respond to Nadine's *no*s and boundaries, using her body language to maintain positive connection, and how to use positive self-talk and motivation in the moment when her desires don't align with Nadine's (see the "Sweet Reminders" portion of the worksheet above).

After taking inventory of her own reactivity to rejection, Sam began practicing several ways to respond to Nadine's *no*s and boundaries that would help her turn toward connection rather than disconnection. Sam practiced verbal responses like the ones listed below in everyday, nonsexual exchanges first in order to make them more automatic to her and reassuringly expected by Nadine. Though these responses aren't complex, the goal is that these constructive verbal shifts will accumulate in Nadine and Sam's relationship over time to make boundaries a normal, welcome part of their life. Below are some examples of positive verbal responses to boundaries that Sam practiced. Feel free to write down some of your own.

- "Thanks so much for telling me."
- "That's good/important info to know about you."
- "I'm so glad you trust me enough to be honest with me."
- "I'm proud of you. Thank you for taking care of yourself."
- "Okay. So, what I'm hearing is [insert your understanding of their boundary], am I getting that right?"
- "Not a problem at all. Do you want to tell me more about this now? Or later on/in couples therapy?"
- "Okay. Do you want to stop here or should we keep doing what we were doing before?"

- "Instead of doing [the thing you were just doing], should we cuddle and watch a movie?"

Sam was also coached to practice not only verbal responses to Nadine's boundary setting, but nonverbal responses as well. To maintain nonverbal connection when discussing boundaries, make sure that your body language supports your understanding of the person's *no*, boundary, or limit, including immediately stopping what you're doing if you're currently sexually engaged, putting physical space between you if appropriate, or maintaining a consistent level of physical connection if appropriate. (For example, if you're snuggled on the couch talking about sex and your partner shares a limit or boundary, rather than physically recoiling in a way that could be received as a punishment, stay connected as consistent with your conversation up until that point.) Other nonverbal signs to be aware of include eye contact, hand-holding, turning away, or sighing in a way that indicates exasperation or disappointment. Generally speaking, matching your nonverbal cues with your verbal cues communicates trust, self-assuredness, and comfort—all important nonverbal messages for your partner to receive in order for them to feel safe sharing their genuine boundaries with you.

Finally, Sam and Nadine practiced giving each other sexual feedback (return to Chapter 8 for tips on how to have a productive sexual feedback conversation) and, in particular, Sam practiced ways to both elicit and respond to Nadine's honest feedback about their sex life (return to Chapter 2 for some additional specific ways to ask for sexual feedback). As I do with many of my clients, I suggested to Sam that she respond to Nadine's sexual feedback with curiosity about Nadine and also curiosity about herself. In her work, Ellyn Bader calls this response practice "Curious, Not Furious"[13]—a handy, rhyming reminder that if we are feeling compelled to automatically and emotionally react to something in the moment, it can actually be more productive and beneficial to try to respond to our partners with questions about their experience of the situation instead (see below for some deeper questions to ask).

"Curious, Not Furious" acknowledges that when a partner says *no* or sets a boundary between something you want and something they just don't, it's normal to feel disappointed, bummed out, or wish things were different. You don't need to react with false excitement to the fact that you and your partner have come to a sexual incongruence. However, it is up to *you*, not your partner, to look at and take responsibility for your side of the street in these interactions. By pouting, pulling away, or taking boundaries overly personally, you risk (intentionally or unintentionally) enticing your partner to caretake your reactions rather than their own feelings as they try to soothe you in order to restore symbiotic harmony. (Remember, that is not the goal.) Instead, practice soothing yourself (using "Sweet Reminders" from the worksheet), unwinding your own rejection-triggered wounds, and responding more productively (for example, "My partner is telling me something about them, not condemning something about me. What can I learn about them right now if I listen?").

With continued erotic differentiation practice by way of taking stock of their own responses, baggage, and triggers nestled within their sex life, Sam and Nadine made continuous progress on their shared goal of bringing ease and chemistry back into their sex life. Sam and Nadine were able to build a new scaffolding of trust and self-reflection around their conversations about their sex life. They learned to ask themselves questions like, "What are my boundaries and why are they important to me?", "What can I learn about my partner in this moment?", and "What do I know about myself that could be making this interaction so challenging for me?" (practicing differentiation) rather than automatically relying on questions like, "Why can't my partner just change already and share all of my same boundaries and desires?" (attempting to revert to symbiosis). Within this erotic differentiation framework, blame, self-pity, and fixation on the other person was minimized and empathy, understanding, and self-growth were maximized, allowing Sam and Nadine to come up with new and more honest solutions to their sex-life conundrums rather than getting stuck in the same old pattern of self-defense and taking offense.

Sam was able to put a stop to her own unhelpful patterns of feeling immediately rejected and downtrodden when what she had hoped would happen in their sex life didn't. Instead, by the end of couples therapy, boundary setting became an open, two-way street between Sam and Nadine that was more of an active flow of conversation rather than an exchange of advances and blocks. With Sam responding to *no* like more of a pro, Nadine was able to manage Sam's disappointed reactions with less of her own defensiveness and with more kindness. Further, she can speak honestly to Sam about what is and isn't working in their sex life, which not only betters the quality of their sex life, but also increases their level of interpersonal intimacy overall. By embracing erotic differentiation in their relationship, the next phase of Sam and Nadine's sex life became passionate, reinvigorated, authentic, revealing, and deeply connected or, as Bader and Pearson would say, full of vitality.

Get to Know Your Partner(s)' (and Your Own) Sexual Self

10 Deeper Questions to Ask or Use as Journal Prompts

Erotic differentiation requires us to deeply know ourselves so that we can hold the structure of our own sexual integrity even when we feel tempted to conform or crumble in our attempts to avoid rocking the relational boat, disappointing a lover, or facing an incompatibility.

Working on erotic differentiation also means welcoming our partners to share *their* sexual selves with *us*, honestly and bravely, so that we can learn how to thrive in difference rather than shirk away from it in a fruitless attempt to maintain symbiosis forever.

The questions below are a good place to start practicing erotic differentiation, either with yourself or a partner. If doing this with a partner, I recommend you ask your partner's permission first ("Can I ask you some questions about your experiences with sex?") and make sure you have adequate time and space for the conversation (like on a long car ride or walk). Always give your partner leeway to decline to answer and remember that even a conversation is a great place to practice consent.

1. When did you discover your interest in _____
_____?
Learning the origin of a kink, desire, or proclivity folds a

person's sexual history into their broader self-discovery story. Listening to your partner's answer to this question can also be a connecting experience as you discuss a vulnerable or exciting memory.

2. What's been your most impactful sexual learning moment?
A person's sexuality often follows a series of *aha* moments. This is a great way to learn about what you or a partner considers especially important or valuable about their sexuality.

3. What was sex education like for you? How did you unlearn what wasn't helpful (or maybe even something harmful)?
Modern sexuality is often informed by overcoming the barrage of misinformation and judgments that we learned when we were younger. This is a great time to reflect on your or a partner's strengths in advocating for who you/ they really are.

4. What was the content of the last piece of erotic media you consumed? What about it really clicked or fell flat?
Erotic content is a common way that people learn new things about their sexual desire, explore their fantasy life, or dip their toes into a new sexual idea. Because of societal shame about porn, this can be a tough one for people to ask about or answer. No need to push the issue if your partner doesn't want to answer or wants to keep this private.

5. When do you feel the most connected to your sexuality? Is it somatic, contextual, relational, environmental?
Sexual desire is often heavily influenced by what's going on around us. This can be a great question to ask if you or you and a partner are exploring issues related to sex drive, such as one of you having a lower sex drive, or one or both of you experiencing a sudden change in sex drive overall.

6. What's a stand-out sexual interaction we've had together? What makes it stand out to you?
What are the moments that send that extra tingle through your sexual body or really kick the sexual chemistry into high gear? Better yet, how can you recreate those moments together?

7. What's a fantasy you return to frequently? Is it one you want to try in real life or would you rather reserve it for your imagination?
Remember, not all fantasies can be realities and some fantasies are best left in the realm of the mind. This question can be a fun way to learn about the biggest sexual organ of all: the brain. It can also be a fun way to spruce up the content of dirty talk or plan your next sexual adventure!

8. Where is somewhere you love being touched? And how?
Everyone's sexual body is unique, which is a huge reason why I advocate for communication as a way to build sexual skill rather than memorizing rote sexual skills to apply to all bodies. This question can help you understand the

specifics of a lover's sexual response and more clearly pave the way toward pleasure.

9. What's one of your biggest turnoffs? What about it shuts you down?
Sometimes this question can remove simple barriers to your best sexual interaction. Or it can highlight a bigger boundary incompatibility that's better addressed sooner rather than later.

10. Is there anything about your sex life or sexuality that you feel like you're grappling with or unsure about? Do you want to tell me about it?
It's rare for people to walk this earth 100 percent confident and sure about everything in their sexual life. Usually, everyone is wondering about something, even if only on occasion. This question can be a deep way to connect about the uncertainness of the human sexual experience. Or it could just stay as a yes-or-no answer without elaboration if this issue is still a vulnerable work in progress.

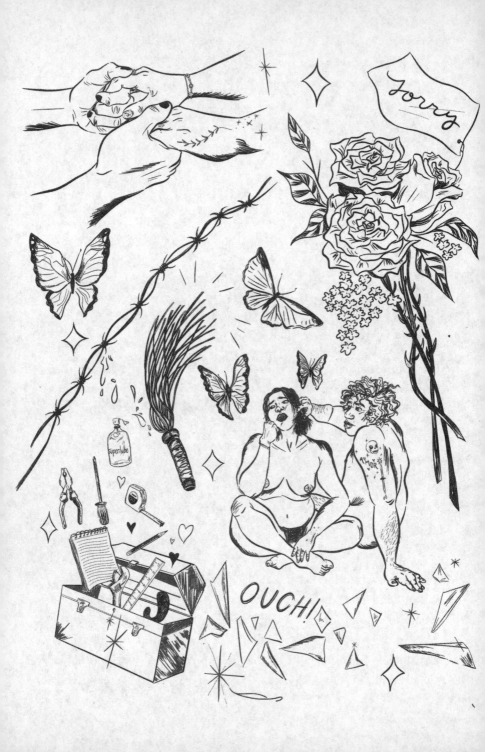

CHAPTER 10

How to Repair a Boundary Mistake

Content note: This chapter mentions sexual assault; however, that is not what this chapter is about. This chapter focuses on everyday, common, unintentional boundary crossings in our sex lives and how to manage them. For more information on sexual assault, violence, and recovery, please see the resource guide.

Accountability, I think, requires taking some agency and courage and moving toward a new pattern of being. It's physically impossible to do that if your body is in a state of shame.[1]
—Lea Roth in "How Shame Can Block Accountability"

How do we turn toward each other to hold this space? And in that turning to each other, we have to say, "I believe you can transform."[2]
—adrienne maree brown in "What Is Transformative Justice?"

We can't fully talk about themes of boundaries, permission, and saying and hearing *no* in our sex lives without talking about what our options are if and when boundaries get unintentionally crossed. The reality is that we are all flawed human beings and, during sex, mistakes will happen despite our best intentions. At some point in your sex life, it is extremely likely that you will cross a boundary and/or one of your boundaries will be crossed. And, for most people, especially those among us who read books like these in the hopes of becoming more consent- and boundary-conscious sexual partners, this is a terrifying prospect.

The scary reality is that no one is immune from causing unintended harm to another person—not even the consent, sexuality, and relationship educators among us. Being a human being means that you likely will unintentionally harm someone in your lifetime. More likely than not, at some point in your sexual life, you will misunderstand a partner's boundary or cross a boundary that you mistakenly overlooked. Or, a partner might retroactively decide that something didn't feel quite right in their sexual interactions with you. It's also definitely possible that you will be on the receiving end of these mistakes, missteps, and realizations that certain moments were harmful. To not acknowledge this here would set us up to believe that we will all always be perfect at boundaries and consent. The truth is, we will not. It would be hypocritical of me to encourage readers to be authentic and human in their sexual experiences while setting the expectation that they will never make a mistake or cross a line.

The realities of violent and intended sexual assault in this country are crushing: 1 in 6 (presumed cisgender) women will experience sexual assault,[3] as will 1 in 33 (presumed cisgender) men;[4] 47 percent of transgender people will be sexually assaulted in their lifetime;[5] and Native American people of all genders, Black transgender women, other transgender women of color, and nonbinary and gender-nonconforming people are highly disproportionately affected[6] by sexual violence in the United States.

Though these intentional, violent, and damaging assaults are a real and global issue, the scope of this chapter will be limited to sexual boundary crossings and misunderstandings that are unintentional and presumed to be relationally repairable. For more information on topics relating to intended harm, such as rape, sexual assault, and long-term patterned abuse, please see the resource guide.

This chapter will specifically address harm done that would fall under 5 on a scale of 1–10 in long-term damage and intensity. Here, we will assume that no intentional physical, emotional, sexual, or relational violence has been enacted by any of the parties involved. An example of what I mean by unintentional harm can be pulled from my experience with Lincoln (described in Chapter 1). Though Lincoln failed to ask my permission before picking me up for an against-the-wall make-out, I did not subjectively experience this as a violent, intended consent violation. I felt awkward, uncomfortable, and embarrassed but I did not feel afraid, intimidated, or in pain.

Subjectively, I experienced this as an overly enthusiastic, misguided, performative gesture of "cool sexiness" that did not work for me. On a scale of 1–10, I would rate the harm done by this encounter as a 1. Lincoln was someone I could trust enough to talk to about it, and I knew he would do his best to correct this unintended mistake in the future if we were to have sex again. However, if Lincoln had done this in a sexual encounter with someone else, that person might have certainly experienced the exact same incident as a harmful consent violation, rating higher on the 1–10 scale.

Other common, unintentionally hurtful boundary-crossing mistakes I've heard from my clients include a partner using certain terminology in overly enthusiastic dirty talk, two partners having different interpretations of "kinky sex," a partner bringing sexual energy into nonsexual contexts, a partner attempting to initiate sex in particular ways that don't feel good to the other partner, or even a partner trying to be overly helpful in trying to remedy the other partner's sex-related issues such as vulvodynia or erectile dysfunction. These are all common ways that we can cross a partner's boundaries in which, though we have not *intended* to be hurtful to our partner, we have still caused emotional, physical, mental, or relational harm to them.

If this topic already has you squirming in discomfort, I don't blame you. Acknowledging that your personal sex life is a place where harm can be done—either by you or to you—is very uncomfortable. But, if we want to ease our discomfort with this topic, and therefore increase the likelihood of doing less harm or knowing how to better repair harm, then we need to talk about it. We are not often taught that harm is inevitable, and we don't talk about the spectrum of sexual boundary crossings enough. Therefore, we are also not taught productive ways to proceed or repair things when harm is done.

Instead, we fall back into black-and-white thinking patterns where anyone who causes harm—even unintentionally—is a bad person. This thinking often drives us (or our partners) to prove that the person who inflicted harm isn't bad, instead of acknowledging the harm done. This usually increases the harm and drives a wedge further between ourselves and our partners instead of keeping us connected as we work through the harm together.

In this chapter, I want to specifically discuss a few alternative ways of navigating these unintentional boundary crossings when all parties involved want to work through that harm together. How can we talk to our partners when they've crossed one of our lines? How can we respond and repair when we've done the line-crossing ourselves? What can accountability look like on smaller and larger scales in our personal, sexual relationships? How do we effectively apologize? And how do the answers to all of these questions contribute to the goal of authentic, pleasurable sex?

Intent versus Impact: What Is Harmful and Who Gets to Decide?

A helpful and popular way to think about harm is along the lines of *intent versus impact*. This means that, although you may not have intentionally wanted to harm your partner, the impact they experienced hurt them emotionally, physically, relationally, mentally, sexually, or otherwise. When we talk about communicating about our boundaries, asking permission, and practicing active consent, the goal is to align our intent with our impact. For example, my partner says they want me to talk dirty during sex. We discuss certain topics they might find hot to talk about during dirty talk. I talk dirty during sex, they're super turned on, I'm super turned on—success! Our intent and impact have aligned!

However, our intent and our impact may not always align. Maybe the next time we have sex, I use a different "dirty" word to describe their vagina than I did the first time. I think this word is super hot, and I'm sure they will think it's super hot, too. But, it turns out, the particular word I chose reminds them of their ex who used to call them that same word in a mean, terrible way during arguments and they find it to be a triggering turn-off that even makes them cry. Of course, my intention was never to conjure up painful memories of their ex or to make them cry during our fun, dirty-talking, sexy times. But that is the impact that my word choice had.

This interaction does not make me a bad person, but it does make me a person who hurt my partner by mistake. Importantly, just because I did not intend to cause them pain does not mean that my partner was not hurt by my words, nor does it mean that they are not allowed to feel hurt. We are two different people with two different thoughts about this word, and we are both allowed to have different experiences of this interaction: mine as some super-casual and fun dirty talk, and my partner's as a triggering name that unleashed painful ideas.

Intent versus impact is a helpful structure to utilize when discussing harm done when boundaries are accidentally crossed because it allows all parties involved to have different experiences. It also means that we can collaborate about how to proceed in repairing the harm done by the incident instead of getting stuck arguing about whose truth is *the truth*.

It also very importantly makes space for the person harmed to have their experience of being hurt validated, believed, and acknowledged. If I were to step on someone's foot accidentally, and they said, "Ouch, you hurt my toe when you stepped on my foot!", I don't get to say, "No, I didn't" or "I didn't even step on your foot." That's not an appropriate response. I do get to say, "I'm so sorry I stepped on your foot and hurt your toe" and, even better, "Can I get you a bag of ice or a Band-Aid? I'll be more aware of where I'm stepping in the future." Furthermore, if I continue to step on this person's foot accidentally, or even if they just don't want to risk a second accidental foot injury, the person I hurt can adjust their boundaries with me accordingly, even if that means breaking off our relationship entirely. (It should go without saying that this is certainly the case if I intentionally try to stomp their toes.) Of course, this is so much easier to think about when talking about stepping on toes, and much more complicated when we talk about harm done during sex.

Shame, Guilt, and Sexual Mistakes

We have all been harmed by the baked-in silence and shame around sex and sexuality. It exacerbates sexual problems and blocks us from easily reaching authentic pleasure. Shame and silence also prevent many of us from being able to access new solutions, safety measures, and conversations about some of the most basic elements in our sex lives (safer sex, talking about desires, saying yes/no/maybe freely), let alone some of the more complicated aspects (harm, crossed boundaries, accountability). Shame is an affective state triggered by a host of emotions (guilt, fear, remorse, anger, arousal, and so on) paired with beliefs about the self ("I'm bad," "I'm weird," "I'm unlovable," "I'm unforgivable").

When we feel shame, our bodies respond physiologically to it.[7] Freezing (shutting down, feeling unable to speak), fleeing (denying one's actions, ghosting, otherwise refusing to engage), fighting (accusing the other person of similar behavior, getting angry as a defense mechanism), and fawning (disingenuously displaying flattery, agreement, or compliance) are all behavioral ways that many of us respond to our deeply rooted desire to rid ourselves of shame. This happens automatically, and without much forethought. By trying to quickly get rid of the shame, we hope to prove—to ourselves and others—that we are not unlovable, unforgivable, bad, or weird, so we can once again be accepted by others, which is a biologically driven need. This is especially true when our actions, behaviors, and shame have threatened our connection to our sexual and romantic partners and, in some cases, to the communities we share with them.

Fortunately, shame and guilt are different. As Brené Brown so cleanly puts it, "Shame is a focus on self, guilt is a focus on behavior. Shame is 'I am bad.' Guilt is 'I did something bad.'"[8] This difference provides us with a path through unintentional harm, accountability, repair, and perhaps even wider transformative justice.[9] The vehicle that carries us through is active consent practice.

Shame and guilt are both necessary guides to the human moral compass. Without them, harm, violence, and disregard for others can easily set in. However, shame, when left unprocessed, prevents us from taking action, thinking empathetically about the people we've harmed, and moving past our own limiting self-beliefs. By contrast, guilt allows us to look at how elements of *who we are* (e.g., power, privilege, mental health, upbringing, circumstance, etc.) have informed *how we have acted*. This framework can help us reexamine our harmful action by looking at it from the lens of guilt rather than shame. Instead of seeing it as a permanent, broken part of who we are, we can instead view it as a regrettable behavior that we can change.

For example, when we look at crossing a partner's boundary through the lens of guilt, we can say, "This is a mistake I made that I feel guilt and shame about, and it's something I can and want to change." By contrast, when the same crossed boundary is viewed through the lens of shame, we may find ourselves thinking, "This is an inherent quality to who I am and there's nothing I can do about it." Guilt allows us to feel more capable and brave, willing to examine, apologize for, take accountability for, and transform that behavior moving forward. In this way, rather than telling ourselves, "I am bad and must remove myself," we can instead say, "I have made a mistake, but I can still have and maintain acceptance and connection."

Sex is a particularly rocky terrain in which to navigate shame and guilt. When we make a mistake, cause harm, or unknowingly trample a boundary in our sex lives specifically, the shame from that error can fuse with any underlying shame we have nestled in other aspects of our sexuality. That combination can magnify and complicate the shame and accountability process.

This umbrella of sexual shame also covers the person who has been harmed. For the partner whose boundary has been crossed, sexual shame can impact how comfortable they feel speaking up about it or how valid or justified they believe their hurt feelings are in the first place. This can look like thinking to yourself, consciously or subconsciously, things like, "If I wasn't into kinky sex this never would've happened" or "This is a natural consequence of having a lot of sex" or "I shouldn't have tried to explore XYZ." I've also heard this shame from clients in terms of wishing they could just be "more chill," "less sensitive," "less activated," or "more relaxed" when their boundaries have been crossed in harmful ways.

But wait! There's another, modern layer of sexual shame that results from unintentional harm in sexual context. I call it the *consent-geniuses layer*. As an independent sex educator who teaches dozens of workshops about consent every year, I am thrilled to see a growing, multi-layered culture of consent blossoming in our classes, on our campuses, in our national vernacular, in our media, and in our personal relationships—sexual, platonic, familial, or otherwise. This beautiful culture of consent can, especially in more sex-positive, LGBTQQIA+, and kink-friendly communities, cast the mirage that "being good at consent" means never making an error or causing harm. These subcultural communities often pride themselves on community care, public accountability processes, and high standards for consent education, practices, and knowledge. These communities are also made of real, fallible humans who may make unintended mistakes or simply not know the community-approved "right" way to do everything.

Though I wish learning a lot about consent resulted in people never making mistakes, sadly it does not. Furthermore, the expectation that this equation is both true and simple is actually not paving the way for acknowledging harm more readily, moving through shame more efficiently, or taking accountability more skillfully. Instead, the cultures of consent that we are building, in sex-positive, LGBTQQIA+, and kink-friendly spaces and beyond, need to include *both* practicing active and various consent processes, *and* making space for repairing screwups (including acknowledgment that repair attempts may need to be made more than once before efforts are deemed satisfactory). I am not saying, "You must love and accept your abuser into your life" or "Oh well, consent violations are just part of the deal," but I am saying, "Expecting people to be consent geniuses is not sustainable, realistic, or kind to ourselves as flawed humans." A successful culture of consent is not devoid of all harm and errors; that standard will never be met. Instead, a successful culture of consent needs to include *all* aspects of the consent process, including various options that the harm-doer and the harmed can choose from when boundaries are misunderstood, misinterpreted, and stepped over.

Eve and Lyndon: Part I
When "Helping" Causes Harm

Content warning: This case example shares a depiction of one couple's struggle with harm caused in their otherwise richly consensual sex life. Feel free to skip to the next section if you prefer not to read it. You won't be missing anything crucial to the learning in this chapter if you do so.

Lyndon and Eve have been dating for several years. Their sex life has historically been robust, exciting, adventurous, and known to include a guest appearance or two by friends and acquaintances. They both have positive relationships to their bodies and sexualities and feel a unique comfort in discussing their desires and boundaries with each other. Eve and Lyndon would be described by their friends as "great communicators" and "sex positive."

Last winter, Eve's sex drive decreased quite a bit. This was a big shift for Eve personally, and for Eve and Lyndon as a couple. Typically very well-matched in their desires for sex, Eve and Lyndon had never had to manage a desire discrepancy in their shared sex life before, and this felt like new, unfamiliar, and unsettling terrain. That's when they made an appointment with me.

The minute our first session started, Eve and Lyndon got to work "fixing their sex life," telling me, "We really think we only need a few sessions to figure this out." They assured me that they had consent, boundaries, and sex positivity down, and what they really needed from me was an outsider's perspective on what the missing piece might be to get their sex life back to normal again.

I generally feel pretty skeptical when couples come in telling me that they really only need to see me for a few sessions so that I can offer a problem fix. Of course, I'm very aware that therapists get accused of stretching out sessions to make money from clients, and maybe even some of them do this. Personally, I think business would be much more successful if I were able to say, "Guaranteed sex life fix in three sessions!" But, typically, that is not realistic or ethical.

In graduate school we are taught to view the problem our clients describe during their first session as the *presenting problem*. The presenting problem is usually the visible icing to the multi-layered cake of other factors and influences going on. These factors can be individual (mental health, trauma, misinformation, body image, self-esteem), relational (communication dynamics, unresolved conflicts, harmful behavior problems), and/or contextual (racism, homophobia, world economics, current political states). Generally, these factors are intertwined, making the presenting problem more complex that it can initially appear. Usually, a three-session Band-Aid isn't going to take your clients far.

In other words, if I had termites in the foundation of my house, I wouldn't just want to patch up the beams those little dudes chewed through. I would want to make sure I got rid of them and learned how to better manage and prevent infestations in the future. So, as a therapist, when a new couple comes in telling me about the presenting problem in their sex life, I don't want to ask, "Where would you like me to affix the Band-Aid?" Instead, I want to know, "Where is the rot? How did it get there? What needs to be done to repair it? And what skills need to be sharpened to prevent it from happening again?" This is the lens that I look through when working with Eve and Lyndon.

Though they both had started couples therapy with me ready to power through a few appointments and be done with it, Lyndon and Eve agreed to slow down the pace so that we could do a little sex life and relationship excavating after I talked a bit about the potential existence of relational rot. In our excavation explorations, Eve shared with me that she had started feeling increasingly depressed the winter she and Lyndon had started having problems, and that her depression combined with their growing relational strife had, understandably, had a negative impact on her desire for sex. Open about most things, Eve had told Lyndon about her depression as soon as she had noticed it that winter, and Lyndon, always a caring partner looking to help, got to work making suggestions, doing research, and buying new products that they thought would jumpstart Eve's sex drive back to normal. These well-intentioned ideas were not the "helpful fix" Lyndon had hoped and only served to further isolate Eve in their relationship.

Though research and suggestions can be a helpful part of repairing an off-kilter sexual connection, they are rarely the full solution. Like most long-term sex partners, Eve and Lyndon had developed a sexual pattern of relating that felt familiar and foundational to their sex life. It's common for long-term sex partners to have a basic framework of sex (I go like this, you do that, we do this, and that's a wrap). This basic framework also becomes the reference point that allows couples to know that they're trying something new or pulling out all of the stops when they do something different. Basic frameworks are great—it's always a good idea to have an ol' faithful routine to turn to that generally satisfies all involved.

However, basic frameworks can also become a bit of a trap, when greater individual or contextual factors shift but each partner's role in the dynamic does not. This can lead clients to feel they are stuck in a rut; I liken it to trying to fit a square peg into a round hole. For Eve and Lyndon, this looked like Lyndon initiating sex just like they always had, taking the leading role and doing "all of Eve's favorite things," and Eve trying to catch up back to "normal" even though her capacity to do so had been drastically lowered by her depression. In this case, the square peg was their typical, favorite sexual dynamic and roles, while the round hole was the current, real-time personal and sexual circumstances of their shared sex life.

By slowing down the pace of our sessions, Lyndon and Eve were able to not only share more contextual and personal information with me, the stranger in the room, but were also able to take some extra time to build trust in the therapeutic process happening between them as partners. With this trust, Eve was able to open up to Lyndon about the harm they had inadvertently caused her by trying to help Eve "go back to normal" and show up to their sex life as she always had. In the context of her current struggle with depression, those efforts were simply not helpful. In fact, Lyndon's nonstop attempts to help were actually harmful to Eve's sexual self-confidence and sense of autonomy because she felt like Lyndon was trying to control her sexual response, pressure her to maintain her typically standard sexual boundaries, and more generally, as Eve put it, "fix her broken self."

Prior to these sessions, Eve had never fully realized or shared how Lyndon's behaviors had impacted her. As she learned more about her experience of their recent sex life, Eve also shared that, in her efforts to not feel broken, she worried that she would let Lyndon down by not "showing up to sex as usual." She would often fake satisfaction while feeling disengaged or not herself. Eve described this as feeling torn between where her brain was actually and where she wanted her body and brain to be, "back to normal again."

Lyndon was, of course, mortified to hear this. They felt awful about their role in creating this cycle, and even worse about accidentally reinforcing Eve's internalized narratives about herself as a sexual partner in Lyndon's life. As a therapist, my role in regard to Eve became making sure she felt safe and empowered to share her story with Lyndon, label the harm done, reassert her boundaries, and determine what she wanted her and Lyndon's next steps to be, if any.

My role in regard to Lyndon became coaching them through processing shame and guilt efficiently so as to not shift the focus too much toward their own internal struggle with these realizations. By doing this, Lyndon was able to show up for, apologize to, and repair with Eve, who, as it turns out, felt open and ready to receive these efforts from Lyndon moving forward.

When You're a Person Who Has Been Harmed

A partner has unintentionally crossed your boundary. Now what?

Only the person whose boundary has been crossed can define the harmful effects of that experience. No one gets to argue it away. Your boundaries are yours and your feelings are yours, and you get to have and experience both in the ways that are authentic to you. If you feel as though a partner has caused you harm or crossed your boundaries, you have a lot of options to choose from.

Here are *some* (certainly not all) of those options; you could choose one, some, or many:

- Talk to a friend about your experience to help you collect your thoughts or feelings, get some third-party validation, and/or seek support.
- Talk to your partner directly . . .
  - ➤ In the moment: "Hang on, I said I did *not* want to use sex toys today."
  - ➤ After sex: "I really liked the rope idea but next time, I'd prefer it if you didn't put it around my ankles—it scares me to have my feet immobilized like that."
  - ➤ Awhile after-the-fact: "Hey, can we check in about our sex life? I've been thinking about a pattern I've noticed in sex with you that I want to change—here it is and here's how I'd like it to change. What do you think?"
  - ➤ A longer while after the fact: "Hi, [Name of sexual partner I haven't talked to or seen in a while], I've been thinking about our past sexual experiences a lot lately and I've realized that some things happened there that actually crossed my boundaries and have been hurtful to me since. I'd love to talk to you about it."
- Adjust your boundaries accordingly. This can include . . .
  - ➤ Temporary adjustments: "Until we can repair this, let's forgo kinky play entirely."
  - ➤ Permanent adjustments: "I don't feel comfortable playing with rope anymore and I'd like to adjust my boundaries accordingly."
  - ➤ Total adjustments: "I no longer feel safe in this sexual dynamic and would like to end it." (Though I *am* saying in this chapter that staying connected through boundary and harm repair is certainly possible, I am by *no means suggesting* that it is always possible nor is it mandatory.)

- Collaborate with your partner to put extra safety checks in place. Such as:
  - Check more often for mutual understanding of a boundary.
  - Increase verbal consent practices.
  - Have longer and compulsory post-sex feedback sessions.
  - Work together in couples therapy and/or separately in individual therapy.
- Utilize a third party such as a trusted friend, mediator, or couples therapist to help you navigate the incident, label harm, and create and witness a repair plan.
- Write a letter to your partner if face-to-face verbal disclosure is too high stakes or challenging.
- Call in[10]: Different from a callout, a call-in is the act of reaching out to someone directly in order to make them aware of their problematic or harmful behavior, words, or actions and how they have impacted you.
- Callout: Callouts have gained speed and impact in a social-media–saturated world and can be understood as publicly denouncing someone's behavior, actions, words, or viewpoints. Though dissecting the complicated modern iteration of "callout culture" is beyond the scope of this book and chapter, this is an option one has and may want to consider, especially if a sexual partner's harmful behavior seems intentional, is meant to cause violent harm, or follows a distinct and unchanging pattern, either with you or with multiple partners. For more reading and considerations on callout culture, head to the resource guide.
- You can also choose to say nothing, especially if you feel that your safety is on the line. In this case, reach out to professionals that can help you leave the relationship or

situation so that you can get to safety[11] (see the resource guide for some recommendations).

As the person whose boundary has been crossed, you also get to decide if a particular violation was indeed harmful to you or if it wasn't. Again, returning to my story of my failed sex date with Lincoln: Although he did not ask my explicit consent before playfully tossing me against the wall, I did not feel harmed by this incident, but someone else might have. If we had chosen to try to have sex together again, I would have corrected course by reasserting my boundary like: "I didn't like being tossed against the wall last time, please don't do that again. And, moving forward, let's talk about any rough body-play options before they're acted on." You also get to decide if you would like to make a repair or if you would not. Or, you might decide that you'd like to attempt to repair the boundary and trust that goes along with it, but during that process you might determine that it's not really working and the relationship may just be permanently damaged.

If you *do* decide that you'd like to talk to your partner about a crossed boundary and harm done, and you also decide that you'd like to move ahead with collaborating on a repair, I'd like to suggest reducing sex-shaming in your discussions. This extra layer of shame typically sneaks its way into these discussions by way of sex- and pleasure-negative social mores. It can be an unhelpful distraction to you and your partner's joint processing of the incident, or can cause someone to equate their non-harmful sexuality as harmful. Instead, if we strive to have a sex-positive accountability conversation, we can further the work to separate shame from guilt and shame from sex, clearing a path for more successful repair and connection. Some suggestions for how to do just this include a sex-positive accountability conversation. This type of interaction:

✘ Doesn't blame someone's fetish, desire, or kink as inherently part of the problem if it isn't.

✘ Doesn't shame someone's desire for sex, whether it's viewed as on the higher or lower end of the spectrum.

✘ Doesn't label consensual sexual experiences with uncalled-for judgment or disgust (i.e., "I can't believe you're even into . . .").

✔ Treats all parties' sexualities and sexual/gender identities as valid and separate from the harmful behaviors done (i.e., never misgenders or questions a person's sexuality as a retaliation again someone who has caused harm).

✔ Resists weaponizing typically shamed aspects of someone's sexual history as proof of harm done (i.e., referencing someone's interest in certain sex acts, relationship structures, number of past sexual partners, or kinks as part of the problem if they are not).

✔ Respects differences in each partner's desires, sexual interests, and what they find to be hot or not.

✔ Aims to maintain ease while talking about sex with one another and also includes tough discussions about harmful behaviors, shame, guilt, and boundaries moving forward.

When You're a Person Who Has Done Harm

You've unintentionally crossed a partner's boundary. Now what?

If nobody is immune to the potential of making a mistake, misunderstanding a boundary, or stepping over a boundary, then nobody is immune to potentially causing harm to a sexual partner—no, not even you or me. If we have caused harm despite our best intentions, we may immediately know it and feel terrible, or we might have no idea and be surprised when someone points it out to us.

If you think that you may have unintentionally crossed a sexual partner's boundary, or if you've just been notified that you've crossed a sexual partner's boundary, there are a few ways forward. If you are looking to process being called out, called in, or otherwise alerted to a pattern of abuse, control, and harm resulting from your behavior, it's time to seek some more advanced and comprehensive resources, some of which can be found in the resource guide.

Responding productively to the realization that you've unintentionally harmed a sexual partner is very important and can be very challenging to do well. Remember, shame can play a big role here, emerging as sexual shame and also the shame of feeling like a bad person. If you've made an earnest mistake in crossing a boundary or harming a partner, and you feel a healthy amount of guilt about it and have the motivation to repair it, you're already on the right path to acknowledgment that you're not a bad person after all; you're simply a flawed human. In fact, the first step to owning up to, apologizing for, and repairing a mistake is to remind yourself that you are not a total piece of shit.

In 2014, Stanford University psychologist Karina Schumann published her research findings[12] that self-affirmation on the part of someone who has caused harm (*transgressors* in her language) leads to better apologies and a higher likelihood of accepted apologies, forgiveness, and relationship repair. She found that positive self-affirmations made transgressors less likely to be defensive in a post-harm conversation, more likely to directly admit to wrongdoings, and included more sincerity and vulnerability in their apologies. Basically, self-affirmation disarms your natural inclination to self-defend (which is not a helpful way to show up to an apology) and bolsters your chances of believing in yourself, feeling strong enough to take accountability for your actions, and creating meaningful repair (which is a *very* helpful way to show up to an apology).

So, if you've made a mistake, crossed a boundary, and caused harm to a partner and they've just told you about it, first take a breath. Though your nervous system may be responding to this news like it's an absolute life-threatening emergency, reacting from this heightened state of perceived threat is not going to go the way either of you would like it to. Instead, take a moment to soothe your own nervous system before responding. Your first response should always be to listen, repeat what you're hearing to check that you've understood, and validate your partner. Remember, you do not need to have the exact same reality. It's highly possible that something you thought was just fine was not fine for your partner, and that is legitimate. You don't need to have had the same experience in order to listen, validate, and stay connected.

Some people who have just been told they've caused harm might want to take a little space to think about, recognize, and collect their intentional thoughts and words before offering a well-rounded, complete apology. Let your partner know if this is you and set clear parameters around that space (24 hours, 3 days, 2 weeks) that the two of you can agree on. This break might be a good time to apply Schumann's findings about the links between successful apologies and self-affirmations. Remind yourself about your core values, how your actions reflect them, and the things you are good at—maybe you're great at a job you love, maybe you're a really supportive friend with a great listening ear, maybe you're a loving parent. Like anyone else, good people make mistakes and cause unintended harm. Write your affirmations down, talk to a friend or therapist, or say them to yourself in the mirror. However, reminding your partner that you are a good person is not appropriate in this moment, so stay on your side of that street.

Now, get ready to apologize.

How to Apologize to Your Partner
A Step-by-Step Option

1. Decenter yourself. Throughout your apology and into your accountability and repair discussions, maintain a focus on your partner's experience, feelings, trepidations, and desired way forward. Although, as discussed above, it can be tempting to defend yourself in order to reassert your goodness and maintain your connection to your partner, this is not the time and your partner is not the audience. A trusted and willing friend, mediator, or therapist is a great place to process your side of this incident, but don't do it here.

2. Say you're sorry. A simple and complete "I'm sorry" is plenty for this first part. Avoid "I'm sorry, but . . ." (justifying your actions), "I'm sorry you feel that way" (shifting blame to your partner's emotional response rather than your actions), and "Sorry this became such a big deal" (minimizing the impact of your actions).

3. Own your actions and mistakes. Showing the other person that you see clearly what your actions were and how they

were harmful solidifies that you, too, understand what happened and therefore are less likely to repeat the same or similar action in the future.

4. Describe what happened. Focus on the behaviors and actions you took and tell your partner in your own words how those actions caused harm. Focus on the facts, not on your intention, inner process, or what you had been hoping would happen. Especially within the context of an otherwise safe and loving relationship, your partner probably already knows that you're not trying to be a monster, so you don't need to defend yourself in that way here.

5. Have a plan. Let your partner know of some ideas you have to repair the situation. It's incredibly important to also ask your partner how they would like to repair the situation, and it can be helpful to bring your own ideas to the table. That way, the onus of fixing your mistake doesn't fall to your partner, but it's important to understand that they might not like or want your ideas. When making your plan, don't forget to zoom out. Most of the time, if we've made an error in our sex lives, it's not just about mishearing a boundary. We are often contextually set up[13] to make these mistakes by complex systems of privilege, identity, sex education, culturally enforced entitlement, and more.

6. Reiterate your commitment to repair. Tell your partner directly that you respect and prioritize their safety and boundaries in your sexual relationship and that you made a mistake. Tell them the specific ways that you plan to mend, work on, or practice the skills you might've been previously lacking in

order to accurately read, understand, check in with, or honor their boundaries in the first place.

7. Take action. The perfect apology is a great start, but it's certainly not enough. If your repair plan includes reading a skills book about kink, consent, sex, and boundaries, then do it. If it involves therapy, an accountability process,[14] or engaging with a mediator, do it. If it involves crafting and practicing new ways of setting and communicating boundaries together in your continued sex life, do it. Don't slack, delay, or make your partner remind you to get to work.

Accountability, at its most basic, is the process of acknowledging, understanding, and taking responsibility for your choices and actions, and for the results and impacts those choices have on others. The interlocking terms of apologizing, accountability, consent, and transformative justice are absolutely relevant to our sex lives and carry with them the weight of pleasure, connectedness, community, acceptance, and justice. It's important to view these terms and the processes they describe not as a box to check but rather as an ongoing skill set to develop, learn more about, and nurture in all of your relationships, sexual or not.

With this continued accountability practice in mind, below are some small ways that we might consistently practice these essential skills as individuals and as sexual and romantic partners proactively rather than reactively.

6 Ways to Practice Accountability in Your Sex Life, Now
Why Wait to Screw Up before Getting Good at This?

1. Talk about sex and relationships more openly with friends. This will help to avoid keeping your sex life in a vacuum, and it will reduce isolation, shame, and stigma. This will also lower the chances that you'll make unchecked sexual choices in a bubble, resist speaking openly about your mistakes, or feel unable to talk through your harmful actions with a trusted community.

2. Frequently check in with partner(s) and friends to ask how you're doing in your relationships with them. This will open regular space for people to tell you if you've made mistakes or hurt them. It will also normalize accountability, apology, and repair.

3. Practice self-reflection in your own behaviors often, whether that's through solo-journaling, therapy, or an accountability buddy system.[15]

4. Don't wait for a big fuck-up. Practice self-reflection and accountability early and often so that if and when you make a big mistake, you have sharpened the skills needed to receive that information, manage your own emotions and reactions to it, and take swift and effective action to apologize, take responsibility, and repair.

5.   Continue your self-education about your own personal relationship to power and privilege. Ignoring or not being aware of the ways power and privilege (e.g., race, gender, finances, social standing, mental health, or physical ability, to name just a few) can foster entitlement increases the chances that you may not see harm you have done or feel justified in doing it. Rather than ignore inevitable power and privilege differences in your partnered relationships, point to them, speak about them, and consider their influence in instances of harm done and boundaries crossed.

6.   If you think you made a mistake, speak up! Don't wait for the person you may have caused harm to do the labor of coming to you first. Be proactive in making apologies and offering repair. Practice the bravery of stepping into that space rather than running from it.

Eve and Lyndon: Part II
Re-empowering Eve with Explicit Permission

In Lyndon and Eve's case, it became clear that after Lyndon apologized to Eve for the harm they had done, the first actionable step was to immediately shift the roles in their sexual dynamic away from Lyndon as "helpful healer" and Eve as "broken person needing fixing." It was crucial here to make sure that Eve felt in control of her physical, emotional, mental, and sexual boundaries and that Lyndon immediately leaned out to give Eve the chance to inhabit this new space on her own terms.

Although this intervention was ultimately directed at their sex life, the first changes happened in their nonsexual life. For example, rather than sending Eve emails and texts of all the helpful resources they had found, Lyndon was given the task of asking for explicit permission before sending a resource or making a suggestion to Eve about anything related to depression and sex. Eve was given the power to say *yes*, *no*, or *maybe* on her own terms, and Lyndon demonstrated to her that they respected these boundaries and heard her loud and clear.

Similarly, Eve and Lyndon took a step back when it came to their physical and verbal sexual boundaries, with Lyndon asking for explicit permission before touching, talking flirtatiously to, or talking about sex with Eve. In therapy, we made sure that both Eve and Lyndon had a written list of examples of when Eve wanted Lyndon to ask permission and made sure that they both clearly understood each other's meaning around these exercises.

After a lot of success in these new roles, Lyndon and Eve did a Yes/No/Maybe List together in order to reboot their boundaries and requests given their current sex-life dynamic. Then, before re-engaging in sex, they practiced integrating these verbal understandings of their new, updated boundaries with intimate touch by doing a few weeks of the boundary and trust repair exercise (found at the end of this chapter).

Through this gradual repair process, Lyndon and Eve were able to take a step back, reestablish boundaries, freshen up their tried-and-true consent strategies, and rebuild trust over time by speaking up clearly, receiving boundaries graciously, responding to boundaries accurately, and giving feedback and adjusting as needed. By taking this scenic route from unintentional harm to sex-life repair, Lyndon and Eve learned new things about themselves, each other, and their shared sex life, and were able to update their sexual routine to be more in line with who they are as individuals and as a couple.

Boundary and Trust Repair Exercise
How to Practice Verbal and Physical Boundary Setting after a Harmful Boundary-Crossing Incident before Getting Back to Sex

Experiencing unintentional harm done by our typically trusted and communicative partner is a jarring experience. Trust may feel shaky, walls may be up, and the willingness to "get back to normal" in your sex life might, understandably, be down. Similarly, if you are the partner who caused unintentional harm, you may be questioning your own formerly trusted abilities to listen to your partner, understand a boundary clearly, and perform effective and active consent checks.

This exercise is all about slowing things down, re-establishing boundaries and trust, checking to make sure boundaries are heard and understood, and opening plenty of space for feedback and adjustments. It is designed to reintegrate the experience of verbally discussing boundaries *during* intimate physical contact before re-engaging in real-time sex as partners again. The goals of this exercise are to: 1) practice verbal and physical boundary skills simultaneously, and 2) gain renewed, lived experience and trust in our partner's and our own abilities to set, respect, check, and honor boundaries, all within a lower-stakes setting than full-on sex.

As with *all* worksheets included in this book, feel free to modify it to be your own or to skip it all together.

Round One

Step One: Decide what physical intimate act you'd like to do together for this exercise. You can also do multiple rounds of this exercise with several different intimate acts. For this example, I'll be using the intimate act of massage.

Step Two: Decide who is initiating touch and who is receiving touch, or if switching, who is going first.
Receiver: Tell your partner all about your massage boundaries—include parts of the body, massage type, length, pressure, no-zones, and accessories (candles, oils, etc.). Include your enthusiastic *yes*es, things you're unsure you want, and your hard-line *no*s.
Initiator: Thank your partner for telling you their boundaries. Tell those boundaries back to your partner in your own words. Ask, "Did I understand those correctly?" when you're done. Do another round of checking your understanding if your partner offers corrections to your original understanding.

Step Three: Start your massage! Set a timer for 15–20 minutes.
Initiator: Ask for consent before starting your massage.

Receiver: Give or deny consent as you see fit. Feel free to say, "*Stop*" at any point, for any reason.

Step Four: Engage in regular, rated feedback.

Initiator: Keep your phone or a clock within view. Ask for direct permission before shifting massage pressure or to a new area of the body. Additionally, roughly every five minutes, ask your partner directly, "How is this feeling?"

Receiver: Rather than respond to your partner with *good* or *bad*, give them a number on a 1–10 scale with 1 being terrible and 10 being amazing. For this round of the exercise, you only need to say the number, nothing else. Of course, if you *want* to say something else, you can and you should. The idea with sticking to the number system for now is to keep you in your body and for your partner to practice giving and receiving feedback in a simplified way.

Initiator: Any time your partner gives you a number, respond with, "Heard [the number they said]." For example, you ask, "How is this feeling?" Partner responds "Six." You say "Heard six." If your partner ever responds with a number lower than five, stop what you're doing and ask them what needs to shift or change.

Step Five: End your massage (when either partner wants to end or when your time is up).

Initiator: Ask your partner to tell you about their massage experience, including things they particularly loved and things they'd like to see change for next time.

Receiver: Let your partner know how things went for you during the massage.

Initiator: Say, "Thanks for letting me know about your experience." If your partner has requested certain things change next time, recap what you heard and tell them your plan for changing it. Ask them if that plan sounds good. If not, make adjustments accordingly.

Round Two

Round Two of this exercise can either be done directly after Round One or can happen the next night, in a few days, or in a week. Decide the pacing that is right for you. For Round Two, do the same intimate act that you did for Round One (so, if you opted for massage for Round One, also do massage for Round Two).

Repeat Steps One, Two, and Three from Round One.

Step Four: Engage in regular, conversational feedback.

Initiator: Keep your phone or a clock within view. Ask for direct permission before shifting massage pressure or to a new area of the body. Additionally, roughly every five minutes, ask your partner directly, "How is this feeling?"

Receiver: This time, instead of responding with a rated number system, respond with your words and directives—"Good," "Bad," "You can apply more pressure," "Can you move to my arms instead of my back?", and so on.

Initiator: Respond to their conversational feedback with what you deem appropriate. For example, if they say, "Good," you can ask, "Do you want me to stay here like this then?" If they say, "Please apply more pressure," increase pressure and check, "Like this?" Any time your partner tells you something isn't feeling good or is feeling less than ideal, stop and ask about what needs to change.

Step Five: End your massage (when either partner wants to end or when your time is up).

Initiator: Ask your partner to tell you about their massage experience, including things they particularly loved and things they'd like to see change for next time.

Receiver: Let your partner know how things went for you during the massage.

Initiator: Say, "Thanks for letting me know about your experience." If your partner has requested certain things change next time, recap what you heard and tell them your plan for changing it. Ask them if that plan sounds good. If not, make adjustments accordingly.

Round Three

Round Three of this exercise can either be done directly after Round Two or can happen the next night, in a few days, or in a week. Decide the pacing that is right for you. For Round Three, do the same intimate act that you did for Rounds One and Two.

Repeat Steps One, Two, and Three from Round One.

Step Four: Engage in regular feedback, however you'd like, whenever you'd like.

Initiator: Check in with your partner for ongoing consent and for feedback any time you'd like to know how things are feeling for them; if a change in pressure, placement, or activity would be okay with them; if you're seeing a nonverbal cue that something might not be quite right; and so on.

Receiver: This time, feel free to give feedback and direction whenever and however you'd like to. If the number system from Round One worked for you, use it. If you'd like to switch to the traditional BDSM color system[16] (green, yellow, red), please do. If you'd like to use verbal, conversational feedback, go ahead!

Initiator: Respond accordingly using the consent and feedback-receiving skills you have, those you've learned about in this book, and the ones you've practiced in Rounds One and Two.

Step Five: End your massage (when either partner wants to end or when your time is up).

Initiator: Ask your partner to tell you about their massage experience, including things they particularly loved and things they'd like to see change for next time.

Receiver: Let your partner know how things went for you during the massage.

Initiator: Say, "Thanks for letting me know about your experience." If your partner has requested certain things change next time, recap what you heard and tell them your plan for changing it. Ask them if that plan sounds good. If not, make adjustments accordingly.

Transitioning to Increased Intimacy and Sex

- Repeat Rounds One through Three as many times as you'd like with as many different intimate actions as you'd like (bathing each other, touching hands, making out, whatever your imagination comes up with).
- When all partners are ready to re-engage in sex, reflect on the following questions to help apply this practice to your

real-time sex life. Share your ideas and considerations with your partner. I recommend going over these questions once, alone, in writing and then again, together, verbally as partners.

- How has our trust in each other changed during this exercise?
- How has my confidence in my own ability to understand, set, and honor my own and my partner's boundaries shifted?
- What kind of feedback style (number system, conversational, timed check-ins, regular feedback sessions, etc.) did we find most effective or helpful and how would we like to integrate that into our sex life moving forward?
- What are some signs that we'd like to put a hold on sex again, back up, and do some more practice of these skills?
- When would we like to check in about how our sex life and these new communication practices are going? (Set a date on the calendar.)

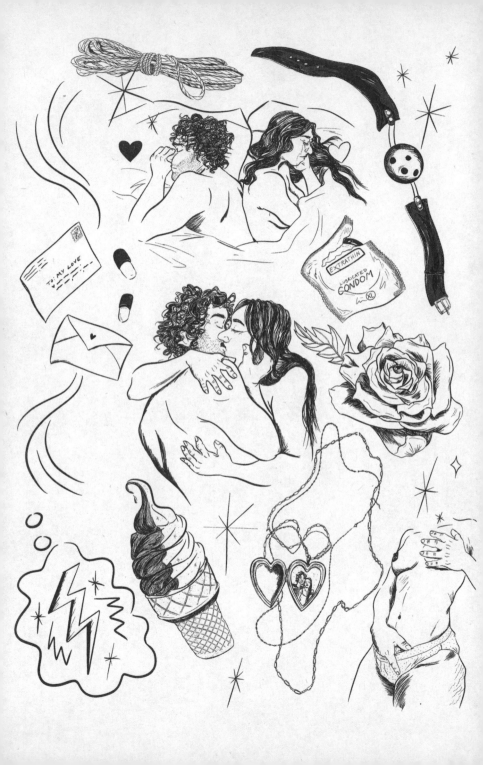

CHAPTER 11

How to Navigate Desire Discrepancies

(When Your Yes Is Their No)

The only way to get out of a gridlock is to move.[1]
—Winifred M. Reilly, It Takes One to Tango

Beyond getting ensnared in a boundary-crossing mistake, there are a few other ways that we may find ourselves feeling stuck or unsure of how or where to move in the complicated landscape of sexual boundaries. This chapter will focus on one of the most common of these stuck places that my clients bring to therapy: a desire discrepancy. Though desire discrepancy is typically defined as one partner having a higher desire than the other partner, there is also a desire discrepancy when one partner has a different desire template than the other (for example, one partner is kinky, while the other is not, one partner is super turned on by anal sex when the other partner considers the booty to be strictly exit-only, or even when one partner wants to be non-monogamous and the other is happier monogamous). Countless sex column write-ins and therapy clients want to know: what do we do when our libidos are mismatched, when her yum is my yuck, or when we just can't seem to get on the same page about what to do behind closed doors?

Of course, the popularity of this conundrum makes sense. If we've learned anything from Chapter 9 and the concept of erotic differentiation, it's that we are all our own unique, little X-rated snowflakes when it comes to sex. There's a pretty low likelihood that two (or more) people with their own thoughts, feelings, beliefs, turn-ons, boundaries, *yes*es, *no*s, and *maybe*s will have exactly complementary desires to one another (and want to spontaneously act on them at exactly the same moment), completely by chance and without discussion. This is true of the casual one-night stand you just brought back to your place and it's also true of the longer-term couple who, over time, have likely changed as individuals (i.e., what you desire, how you desire it, and what you want) and as a couple (i.e., what our chemistry is like, how we initiate and move through sex, what sex means to our relationship). Your chances of having a desire discrepancy crop up during your time on this planet as a sexual being are certainly higher than your chances of never facing a desire discrepancy at all. And grappling with a desire discrepancy can certainly be a sticky little pickle to find yourself in, especially one that pops up in an otherwise satisfying relationship.

Most advice columnists and relationship experts might tell you that, in these and in all relational dynamics, compromise is key. I say that compromise is overrated. In fact, when it comes to consent-based, pleasure-focused sexual relationships, compromise can actually be pretty harmful and icky. Instead, I recommend a return to the erotic-differentiation model from Chapter 9 and all it can offer to navigating desire discrepancies in all kinds of sexual relationships. This is exactly what we'll do in this chapter, and here's why: When compromise is assumed to be the key, the individuals in the relationship are told to modify their own boundaries and desires in order to preserve the relationship itself. In the case of a desire discrepancy, this might look like "I'll try getting tied up if you try wearing a strap-on" or, far more commonly, "I'll have more sex with you than I want to in order to keep the marital peace even though I'm not into it." In this model, maintaining the relationship is the primary goal to be met at almost all personal cost.

Conversely, when we address desire discrepancy within the erotic-differentiation model, the bull's-eye of the target is not automatically set on saving the relationship no matter what. Instead, the goal is for each individual to get diamond-level clarity about their own boundaries and what's important to them as a unique sexual person. This can include understanding which boundaries you're willing to explore, challenge, or flex; what you are and aren't willing to experiment with or try; which sexual experiences and desires are crucial to your sexual self-expression; and can even include compromise *if you choose it* (more on that later). The erotic-differentiation model, on the other hand, does not center compromise as the only or even the preferable solution, and it certainly doesn't set it as the default. Compromise is great when it means "I'll cook dinner if you do the dishes," but it's not good in a situation like "I guess I'll do anal if you'll agree to more foreplay." That doesn't work and can leave partners feeling icky.

The "Compromise Is Key" Model:

- Frames sexual acts and experiences as transactional currency.
- Leads to lukewarm or even undesired sex for at least one partner at least some (if not most) of the time.

- Involves one person conforming to the other person for a short period of time in order to check off a box or restart a timer.

- Reduces self-definition or genuine self-exploration.

- Encourages your partner to (dis)engage with your sex life in a false, suppressed, or otherwise disingenuous way.

- Speeds to a logistical solution rather than peeling back the layers of meaning underneath each person's sexual experience.

- Encourages partners to make compromises or shift their boundaries without first fully considering what it would mean to them personally if they were to do so.

- Promotes a "taking one for the team" mentality of sex, which (I've said it before and I'll say it again) is an icky way to have sex.

- Deprioritizes boundaries, communication, pleasure, and consent.

The Erotic-Differentiation Model:

- Is rooted in honesty, self-definition, and, you guessed it, the broader concept of differentiation.

- Encourages each partner to make a thorough and genuine assessment of what they are and are not willing to do, try, experiment with, or explore *before* they take action toward a compromise or solution.

- Is an active- and informed-consent model of navigating difference.

- Connects each individual person to their core values, beliefs, and limits around sex, desire, relationship, and sexual expression.

- Brings partners to a solution that is rooted in genuine pleasure, self-knowledge, and individual integrity.
- Prioritizes the person before the relationship, making for a longer-lasting, more authentic connection if the relationship is to continue and sheds light on an inherent incompatibility or deal-breaking sexual difference if it is not.
- Allows each partner to decide what is or isn't crucially important for them to have as part of their sex life (i.e., carefully answering the question "What are you willing to not have in your sex life?" in order to make an informed and willing sexual concession).

Having a sex life centered around active consent, authentic pleasure, and secure boundaries can't just be the case when we're on the same page about what we want out of sex and relationships. Personal and relational integrity also needs to hold true when we inevitably come up against a difference in desire or a clash in boundaries. Navigating desire discrepancies with erotic differentiation rather than compromise is an informed consent model of difference management, one that sharpens each individual's boundaries, explores why these boundaries are important, and guides each person to an authentic solution without harmfully compromising their own core values, sexualities, deepest desires, or limits. This is why I frequently use this approach in my therapy practice to help clients traverse inevitable difference along the entire spectrum of casual sexual relationships (as we'll see below with my client Mia) and more serious and committed relationships (as we'll see when we return to Brandon and Thom from Chapter 8).

Mia and Dan: Erotic Differentiation and Disparate Sexual Boundaries

We can't talk about erotic differentiation (or differentiation as a broader concept) without talking about anxiety. Even if we're a *totally chill person*, relational anxiety can sprout up easily in the cracks made when a formerly symbiotic relationship has just tripped over its first incompatibility. In the clients I've worked with, I've seen many iterations of this anxiety-provoking incompatibility: one partner has started deprioritizing sex post-baby while the other partner continues to hold it to the same level of importance; one partner wants to introduce sex toys while the other partner thinks their bodies alone should be enough; or an incompatibility can crop up early on, like with my client Mia who, in her twenties and on dating apps, has found that most people she's been dating want to move sex along at a much faster pace than she does and she isn't sure what to do about it. In all of these scenarios, anxiety is likely to creep in no matter which character you are in any given scenario: the partner interested in sex toys doubts her "need" for them once she sees her partner's reaction to the suggestion; the partner who doesn't want the sex toys is concerned about their level of sexual ability and wonders if they'll be replaced by a vibrator; the higher-desire partner worries that she'll never be sexually satisfied again; and the lower-desire partner chastises himself as he thinks, "What's wrong with me? Shouldn't I want sex more?"

In Mia's case, she's worried that she's "unnaturally prudish" for her peer group and thinks she should just "catch up already." With this narrative already lodged in her mind, she begins dating a new guy about a year into our therapeutic work together, which has so far been focused on helping Mia manage the stresses of school, social life, and family. Mia met Dan on a dating app and they had just been on their third date when Mia came in for her session that week, already in tears before she had even landed on my office's couch. "I've already had like three meltdowns today," she says, attempting a smile and sipping her iced coffee instead. Mia hasn't been much of an in-session crier during our time together, so I'm a little concerned and definitely curious. "Oh yeah? What's going on?"

Mia: You know that guy Dan I've been dating?
Me: The art major guy?
Mia: Yeah. He sculpts. Anyway, I feel like I'm doing this whole dating thing wrong with him but I, like, don't know how to stop. Every time I go over there, I tell myself I'm not going to go any further in the hooking-up realm, and then I just do. He's not pressuring me or anything, he's great, and we're having so much fun otherwise, I just don't know what I'm doing. It's making me feel really bad about myself.

Mia is 24 years old and relatively sexually inexperienced. Though neither Mia nor her parents have a no-sex-before-marriage policy, Mia does have slightly more conservative sexual values than her friends and has always moved at a slower clip than her peers when it comes to sexual and romantic relationships. Instead, she's preferred to focus her early adulthood on her studies, friendships, family, and creative endeavors, all of which have made her very happy and fulfilled. However, now moving further into her twenties, Mia has begun to take more of an interest in dating, hooking up, and sex but so far has felt ill-equipped to do so.

We had discussed Mia's sexual values, boundaries, wants, limits, and dating life as she began to create a vision for what she wants her emerging sex life to look like during our sessions. This was challenging for Mia at times because her peer group has largely been raised in the age of the internet, dating apps, sex positivity, hook-ups, and an overall faster pace between meeting, dating, and having sex (or, at least, that is her perception of her peers). Dan confirms Mia's perception by assuming a casual attitude about sex and by presuming that Mia shares the same attitude about sex as he does. In actuality, Mia has recently gained the new clarity for herself that she really values emotional connection before sexual connection and that she wants to be in an exclusive, defined relationship with someone *before* she has sex with them. Judging by his behavior alone, this stands in contrast to what Dan's values around sex are and, because Mia's unsure how to manage this difference in the moment, she has found herself collapsing her own values and boundaries more often than she would like in favor of preserving the Classic Mood and its pal, symbiosis. This collapsing is exactly what is causing Mia distress—not her more conservative values, not Dan's casual sexual attitude, and not even the desire discrepancy itself—but the ease with which Mia finds herself abandoning her boundaries in favor of appearing "normal" or fitting in. As we discuss this further in therapy, we learn that Mia's lack of available options in *responding* to this desire discrepancy between them is the culprit that has made their sexual dynamic so quickly problematic.

A desire discrepancy of any kind is a natural disruption to the smooth sameness of the symbiotic stage (that la-la-land stage covered in Chapter 9) because it is, at its core, an unignorable difference. When it comes to a (predictable) rupture in the walking-on-sunshine symbiotic stage of a new relationship, it's normal to feel anxiety, worry, fear, or even judgment, anger, and irritation. These emotions are natural responses to our fears of being left, abandoned, replaced, or judged (see Chapter 7) as we fear that we are no longer the same as or complementary to our partners, signaling an inevitable loss of the relationship in question. When we feel these emotions and fears, we experience anxiety, an uncomfortable state of being that most people try to quickly resolve by way of returning to the way things were. In our "compromise is key" brains, we rush to point to "the problem" so that we can find a quick "solution." And in the "compromise is key" model, this solution tends to be—yep!—compromise.

However, compromise does little to actually solve a desire discrepancy and can often do more harm than good to both the individuals involved and the relationship itself. When the symbiosis bubble is popped by something like a desire discrepancy and we go searching for a problem to fix, we tend to do one of two things. One thing that's likely to happen is that we turn inward with self-blame ("I should sleep with my wife more if I want to be a good husband," "I should just be happy with what our bodies can do and not want to include toys," "I should take one of those quick-fix supplements to increase my libido and then we won't have this problem"). Otherwise, we are likely to turn outward and blame our partner ("If he exercised more he'd probably want sex as much as I do," "She doesn't need a vibrator, she just needs to learn how to climax naturally," "I wish they would just stop rejecting me so much").

This instinct to reach for self- and other-blame comes from our efforts to banish the "problem" that we believe is causing relational tension so that we can stop feeling anxious and go back to la-la land already. However, when we do this, we either internalize the problem as "something wrong with me" or we look at it as "something wrong with my partner." This establishes an unhelpful process that does little to solve the actual problem and instead creates shame, self-doubt, and silence in our sexual relationships rather than openness, curiosity, acceptance, and progress. This response of blaming ourselves or our partner often leads us to the default "compromise is key" model, where we seek a quick fix by modifying our own behavior, or pushing our partner to modify their behavior. Rather than creating a sustainable and authentic solution, this method often creates disconnection, resentment, and chronic self-editing. In Mia's case, she has gone the self-blame route, and believes that there's something wrong with what she considers to be her unusual desire for an emotional connection before sex. It has become a "problem" she has fruitlessly tried to "fix" by pushing herself beyond her own limits and collapsing her boundaries.

This subconscious instinct to blame ourselves or others, collapse our boundaries, or push past our authentic limits is also causing distress for our longer-term couple, Brandon and Thom, who we met in Chapter 8. It's not just new relationships that can get trapped in a symbiotic stage or suffer from the "compromise is key" mentality as partners struggle to thrive in the differentiation stage. Though new relationships do tend to be blissed out on symbiosis, *new* and *symbiotic* are not synonymous. Even older, tried-and-true relationships can hit the skids of differentiation in unexpected ways. The longer we are in a partnership with a person, the more likely it is that we will change and evolve—both as individuals and as partners, requiring us to once again practice differentiation when we do. This is because personal and dynamic evolution can trigger the relationship itself to evolve out of a comfortable symbiosis and into a new stage of differentiation, a process that (in my opinion, which not all therapists share) can happen more than once as we swing in and out of symbiosis and differentiation within the various layers and life stages that create any given relationship over time—sexual, romantic, family-building, financial, cohabitational, and more.

Brandon and Thom: Erotic Differentiation and Mismatched Libidos

Brandon and Thom, who we were introduced to in Chapter 8, first started their couples therapy work with me after struggling with their sexual connection for the last three years. Brandon, identified as the higher-desire partner, was feeling downright downtrodden as their formerly fiery sex life became practically nonexistent. Thom had identified himself and his lowered libido as the problem that needed fixing. As you can imagine, beating yourself up about your diminished sex drive does little to turn it back on, and Brandon's growing despondency about being repeatedly rebuffed by Thom certainly wasn't helping matters.

In Chapter 8, we learned about some of Thom's personal barriers to his own sexual desire, including never having had the opportunity to discover his sexual self with men beyond what he had experienced with Brandon, one of his first-ever male lovers. Though previously, Thom and Brandon had happily created a symbiotic stage that consisted of Brandon taking the experienced lead, Thom had outgrown this role and, when he did, his sexual desire began to stumble. As a result, he and Brandon began to struggle in earnest with their own differentiation stage.

Thom began to remove this barrier to his sexual desire by exploring new erotic interests and taking charge to bring them back to his relationship with Brandon. Meanwhile, Brandon learned how to dissolve the caked-on resentments that had built from what he experienced as consistent sexual rejection from Thom. He practiced how to better manage his own responses to Thom's present-day *no*s and boundaries (just like Sam did in Chapter 9). Thom and Brandon began to have compulsory sexual feedback conversations about both their new and old sexual experiences together (see page 281) and they began a tried-and-true therapy technique called *externalizing the problem*.

Externalizing the Problem

Externalizing the problem is a therapy technique rooted in narrative therapy,[2] a style of therapy that focuses on readjusting the stories we tell about ourselves, our relationships, and our problems in order to find new ways to view them, cope with them, and overcome them (might ring a bell from Chapter 5). This technique is one way narrative therapy can help a person feel more powerful than their problems. The process of externalizing the problem does this by pinpointing the ways people overidentify with their problems, and then working to separate the person from the problem. This leads to: 1) helping the person feel more confident that they can indeed change (instilling hope) and 2) making the problem appear to be more malleable and less permanent.

The technique of externalizing the problem is primarily done through language. By adjusting how we *talk* about ourselves and our problems, we can adjust how we feel, think, and act in relation to those problems. For example, imagine that you have a splinter lodged in your right thumb, so it really hurts when you text. If you were to overidentify with your problem it might sound like "I'm a bad texter." Instead, if you were to separate yourself from your problem it might sound like "I have a splinter in my thumb, so it hurts when I text. There are a lot of other ways I can communicate with people including talk-to-text or a good ol' fashioned phone call. Once I'm able to remove this splinter, it'll hurt less when I text so I'll be more likely to pick it up as a communication tool again. This splinter is really the problem, not me. Let's think of some ways to remove it or work around it."

In a mental health context, specifically, overidentification can sound like "He's a depressed person" rather than "He is a person struggling with depression," or "This just isn't working" rather than "When XYZ problem occurs, our relationship really suffers." For Brandon and Thom, Brandon would say, "Maybe we're just not sexually compatible" and Thom would say, "I'm just not horny enough to satisfy Brandon, I guess." And, as their therapist wanting them to externalize the problem, I say, "So, what do you each do when The Mismatch arrives in your bedroom?"

Although this question might make it seem like I have truly not been paying attention, it's actually an intentionally overexaggerated personification of Brandon and Thom's presenting problem. Though it may be true that Brandon is inherently more interested in having sex more often than Thom, or it may be true that Thom is currently less interested in sex than he has been in the past, these separate experiences are actually less problematic than the way Brandon and Thom are currently *relating to the problem*.

Though Brandon can find ways to take care of his own high desire (masturbation solo and/or masturbation with Thom's willing assist such as via sexting), and Thom can move barriers to his lowered libido, these things are *parts* of the solution, not the *entire solution*. These individual pieces of the work will be more effective when done in conjunction with externalizing the problem. Traditionally, the first step to doing this is to identify and name the problem as the problem—not as a permanent feature of either partner ("I'm just not horny enough") and not as a permanent feature of the relationship itself ("Maybe we're just not sexually compatible"). I chose the name The Mismatch just to kick us off. In narrative therapy theory it's important that the clients name their own problem, and this is just as well because, as it turns out, Brandon and Thom had misheard "The Mismatch" as "Ms. Match." Having a great sense of humor, they decided to roll with this ultra-personified and punny version of their woes. (Have I mentioned how fond I am of my clients?)

Your Turn: Name That Problem!

1. Write your problem out in one sentence:

2. Rewrite that sentence separating you (the person/people/
sex life/relationship) from the problem:

3. Now, name that problem! (For example, Ms. Match).

Now that we have a name, we've got a common enemy. Because Ms. Match is not Thom, is not Brandon, and is not their relationship, we can be harsher in our critiques, acknowledge the damage she's done, reduce Brandon and Thom's blame and shame, and gain a new view of possible solutions. Most importantly, Brandon and Thom can band together to defeat her unwanted effects on their sex life. Because narrative therapy and externalizing the problem are all about retelling an old, familiar story in a way that breathes new life and possibility into it, we start with a narrative therapy technique called an *externalizing interview*[3] about Ms. Match before we attempt to generate new solutions. This helps Brandon and Thom reconfigure their thinking about their mismatched libidos as a common issue that the two can work together to solve. It also recasts them as characters in their story that are being influenced by the third entity in their relationship, Ms. Match. This externalizing interview also helps them think creatively about the situation they find themselves in with Ms. Match rather than keeping them stuck in their original stories that have implied that either one of them is broken, too much, or not enough, and that their sexual relationship may just be doomed to fail.

Below are the questions I asked Brandon and Thom. They include some common externalizing questions that may be posed by a narrative therapist looking to help their clients separate themselves from their problem story, and I encourage you to answer them for yourself using the new, externalized, named version of your problem.

Externalizing Interview Questions

- How long have you been noticing Ms. Match?
- What effect does Ms. Match have on your sex life?
- Does Ms. Match impact other areas of your relationship? How?
- What do you think about the effects Ms. Match has on your sex life and relationship?
- How do you feel when Ms. Match is present?
- How do you act or respond to your partner when Ms. Match is present?
- How does Ms. Match inform your thoughts and feelings

about yourself? About your partner? About the relationship? About your sex life?

■ Brandon, how do you imagine that Ms. Match makes Thom
feel, think, or act as the "lower-desire" partner?

■ Thom, how do you imagine that Ms. Match makes Brandon
feel, think, or act as the "higher-desire" partner?

■ Brandon, how does Ms. Match try to convince you that you
and Thom just aren't sexually compatible?

■ Thom, how does Ms. Match try to tell you that you're "just
not horny enough" to be Brandon's husband?

■ Are these effects of Ms. Match acceptable to you?

■ How would you prefer to act or respond to Ms. Match?

By sharing their answers to these externalizing questions together in session, Brandon and Thom make some important, dust-
clearing shifts in their couples therapy work:

■ They each get to hear the other person express empathy
for their position and take their perspective.

■ Rather than continue to argue about the problem, they
take the time to express and hear the deeper and more
vulnerable feelings behind the problem (fear, inadequacy,
hopelessness, etc.). This helps them each identify just how
hard this problem has been on them as individuals and
helps soften any resentments or frustrations that have
built up toward the other over time.

■ They break any silence and stalemating to bring the
problem to light.

■ Each person is able to reframe their own self-sabotaging

thoughts as valid ripple effects of the problem at hand
that are being caused by outside forces, not internal, permanent traits.

- Despondency, giving up, and ideas that "maybe this just
  isn't going to work" are replaced by hope, motivation,
  and "maybe we could try XYZ."

- And, my personal favorite jumping-off point for our next
  sessions, both Brandon and Thom begin to view their
  problematic patterns around this issue from a bird's-eye
  view, making these behavior patterns more malleable to
  change.

This last bullet point helps Brandon, Thom, and me continue
their work on the level of actionable steps each one of them can
take to reshape the problem and reduce the power Ms. Match has
had over their thoughts, feelings, sex life, and broader relationship. And here we come to the last of our interventions that can
be taken by partners who are struggling with the very common
issue of a desire discrepancy: conscious compromises.

Conscious Compromises Are Actually Key, Though

In the context of any desire discrepancy, in order to move away
from the knee-jerk "compromise is key" model and toward erotic
differentiation, we need to (counterintuitively) refocus on ourselves first so that we fully understand our contribution to the relationship's problem cycle before heading into possible solutions.
This can look like getting to know your boundaries and what
they mean to you and exploring the deeper self-expression and

validation you get from the sex acts you love. It can also look like sharing and listening to your own and your partner(s)' answers to the questions listed in the "Get to Know Your Partners' (and Your Own) Sexual Self" box from Chapter 9 or the "Externalizing Interview Questions" in this chapter. Basically, rather than compromising wants and needs willy-nilly in order to find some sort of faux "fairness" that looks good on paper ("I'll do X if you do Y"), a couple navigating desire discrepancy with erotic differentiation as their guide will do things on purpose in a way that *feels* good off paper, in practice. By doing so, each member of the couple can be sure that the other person is agreeing to things, letting go of things, or shifting their *maybe*s to *yes*es, or their *no*s to *maybe*s, in a way that is informed, intentional, consensual, and less likely to end in regret, resentment, or *disingenuous* compromise.

As we've seen throughout this book, in most sexual relationships, it is unlikely that each person's level of desire for sex (frequency of sex itself, libido level, time thinking about and talking about sex, etc.), preferred flavor of sex (rough, vanilla, kinky, sensual, gentle, emotional, casual, etc.), and desired content of sex (specific sex acts, positions, roles, etc.) will be perfectly aligned. It's likely that you will run into a desire discrepancy at some point and it's likely that the solution to that desire discrepancy, if you are to stay together, is going to include some kind of compromise. "But wait!" you might say, "Didn't you just spend pages and pages convincing me that the 'compromise is key' model is bad advice?" Why yes, I did and it is. Jumping right to a compromise without moving through a process of erotic differentiation is an unhelpful, questionably consensual move. However, coming to a point of conscious compromise after you've looked carefully at your boundaries and values—and the level of importance of the desire you're having a discrepancy about—is a necessary part of most sexual relationships. So, what is a conscious compromise and how do you make one?

A conscious compromise is a compromise that is made willingly after honest self-reflection about what the compromise will mean to you, to your partner, and to your relationship. You must bravely ask, "How important is this issue to me?", and answer truthfully, to yourself and even out loud to your partner. A conscious compromise involves being able to *both* tell your partner what your side of the desire discrepancy means to you *and* why and how, specifically, you are willing to flex your boundaries around it. For what should be obvious reasons, it's crucial that this is done with your fullest consent and also without guilting, shaming, or otherwise using your compromise as leverage over your partner to get what you want later on, about something else. This is also a process that may require most of us to get more comfortable living with the unknown ("What will happen, over time, if we make this compromise?") and will be made far easier the better we are at erotic differentiation ("I'm willing to look at, identify, and advocate for my own needs and boundaries even in the face of difference or potential conflict/separation"). Here's how this might look for some of the partners we've met in this book.

In Chapter 8, Jack worked in therapy to identify and label his dislike of receiving blow jobs and build self-acceptance and self-advocacy around this boundary, a skill he set out to utilize in his future dating life. After doing this, he started dating a new woman, Julia. Jack and Julia clicked on every level except for one: giving blow jobs is her number-one turn-on. She *loves* it. Jack, having just done all of this work to solidify his *no* to blow jobs in therapy, feels strongly that he shouldn't cave to a new girlfriend's desire. However, he also wants Julia to feel fully satisfied in their sex life and is worried that if she can't explore her eroticism in this way, that she will ultimately be unhappy with their sexual relationship and even perhaps end it.

To work toward a solution, Jack decides to "talk about talking about the thing" (Chapter 7), and addresses this desire discrepancy head on. In this conversation, he will share with Julia his concerns that if he starts talking to her about why this desire is important to her, that, in order to make her happy, he will eventually just give up his boundary in a way that doesn't feel good to him. In this conversation, Jack discloses to Julia the work he had just done in therapy around this exact issue. Having not previously known about all of the hard work Jack had put into this boundary, Julia emerges from this conversation feeling strongly that it's more important that Jack maintains this hard-won boundary than it is for her to have blow jobs be part of her current sex life. Instead, Jack and Julia take a deeper dive into what it is about blow jobs, exactly, that is so erotically charged for Julia. For her, she shares, the consensually submissive act of giving pleasure in this way is a huge turn-on. With this information, Jack and Julia decide to experiment with a variety of sex acts and sexual flavors that conjure up these similarly submissive, pleasure-giving feelings and agree to revisit the blow job issue once their relationship is more established and/or if Julia ends up feeling strongly that she needs that sex act to be a part of her life, whichever comes first.

Kira, who we also discussed in Chapter 8, surfaced from her divorce and years of sexual dissatisfaction with a new confidence and bravery in exploring her latent kinky nature. In therapy, she worked to establish boundaries that honored this kinky self and allowed her to safely explore prioritizing this aspect of her sexuality. As part of that boundary setting, Kira decided she only wanted to engage in sexual relationships that were kinky by design, casual, and with partners who were previously experienced with kink.

Later, she hit it off with a woman she met at a bookstore. Having no idea if this person was kinky or not, Kira asked her out for coffee and they continued to hit it off over several lattes. Staying true to herself and her boundaries, Kira kicks off the sexual part of their relationship by talking about her boundaries, needs, wants, and likes first, including her preferences around kink. Though this woman has never explored kink before, she's excited and open to the prospect. Kira decides that in this context, she's willing to flex her boundary about previous kink knowledge and shifts the boundary to having non-kinky (vanilla) sex be part of their dynamic until more trust is built between them, at which time they'll both attend some workshops and educational/social kink events to build their knowledge and kinky dynamic together, as they go. Kira reasserts that it's crucial to her to have kink be a part of her sexual life and so they both agree to reassess this issue as they go, leaving room for this new partner's self-discovery about whether or not kink seems right for her as she learns more about it herself.

Cam and Brit briefly appeared in Chapter 7 when Cam broached the topic of non-monogamy. Cam has decided that she wants to explore non-monogamy, which would be a shift in her and Brit's previously monogamous relationship. In their discussions about it, Brit becomes clearer that they are more comfortable with and more interested in monogamy, and they just don't feel like "a non-monogamous person." Brit agrees to give it a try for the sake of wanting to maintain their otherwise happy relationship but for a limited period to see how it feels. Brit and Cam agree to specific boundaries of their open relationship trial run and set a date to rediscuss this issue and any new thoughts or feelings that have come up during that time. After a couple of challenging months, Brit feels more sure in their desire for monogamy and Cam in her desire for non-monogamy, and the couple decides to part ways in order to keep themselves available to the relationship style they each truly want.

Brandon and Thom were able to externalize the problem of their Ms. Match and were able to reduce blaming themselves and each other, and become more intimately connected through the therapy process itself. Thom and Brandon create a new way of relating to their libido mismatch that is less loaded, less toxic, and more connected. The sexual spark reignites for them both and a new sexual dynamic emerges as Thom initiates more and Brandon controls less. They communicate more, and each partner respects their own and each other's desire levels as a lovable part of their relationship that they collaborate to maintain throughout their long-standing marriage.

The only way to reach a conscious compromise in your sex life or relationship is to take the path of erotic differentiation to get there. This includes brave (and sometimes blunt) inventory of your own and your partner's boundaries and desires and what specifically makes them so important and valuable to each of you. Just like you don't sell a house without first getting it properly appraised, don't give away what is sexually true for you without knowing what exactly it is you are agreeing to let go of, experiment with, or explore, and for how long. To help you in this careful appraisal are some key questions to ask yourself and talk about with your partner before jumping to the conclusion of compromise. Not every question will fit every scenario, but each should be considered with ongoing consent and the evergreen ability to change your mind at any time.

Questions to Ask Yourself before Making a Conscious Compromise

- How important is this issue to me? What would it mean to me to have this desire or boundary compromised in some way?
- What are the benefits to me, to my partner, and to our relationship if I make this compromise?
- Is my hesitance/resistance to making this compromise based in any kind of lingering sexual shame, phobia, or self-judgment that is unnecessarily holding me back?
- Does making this compromise violate any of my fundamental boundaries, values, or limits?
- How will I know if this compromise isn't working for me? What are some signs to look out for?
- Would it be helpful to have a time limit or check-in date around this compromise? (For example, let's try opening our relationship for three months and then reassess how it's working for us.)
- Do I trust that my partner can and will reassert their needs if this compromise isn't working for them? Do I trust myself to do the same?
- When I think about making this compromise, what do I feel in my body and where do I feel it? What is this gut instinct telling me?
- Are there ways this compromise could be made in smaller installments? Would that help me feel more sure about it? (For example, I'd like to try XYZ sex act twice and then reassess if I'd like to keep doing it.)

- Do I feel safe and comfortable saying "no" to this proposed compromise either now or in the future once we've started enacting it?
- Do I need more time to think about this compromise before I agree to it?
- Is there anything else I need to ask myself, my partner, or explore further before I agree to this compromise?

Advice like "compromise is key" pressures many people to sacrifice important parts of their sexual selves, and it intertwines with the external messages we get about pleasure and sex. Let's return to Mia and her attempts to navigate her desire discrepancy with Dan as best she can with the resources she has. Like many people, one of Mia's deep, interpersonal goals is to be accepted, which, in the context of her relationship with Dan, looks like doing whatever she can to feel relationally successful by making their otherwise lovely connection work. As we've seen, there are several reasons why Mia has instinctually tilted toward staying quiet, editing herself, denying her own needs, and assuming that "this is the way sex goes [for women]" all the while pushing herself to keep Dan's sexual pace (see Chapters 1, 2, 4, and 6). Because of all of these intersecting personal, social, and contextual reasons, Mia has identified *herself* as the problem rather than looking at the *dynamic* between the two of them as the real, workable issue.

In the "compromise is key" model, the quickest solution is compromising her own core sexual values, beliefs, and boundaries as she internally pressures herself to conform to Dan (and their hoped-for relational harmony). She assumes that he is already compromising by moving at her "unnaturally slow pace." These automatic thoughts and assumptions block Mia from experiencing her most pleasurable sex life, deprioritize consent and authenticity, and prevent Dan from getting to know the real Mia. The effects of all of this on Mia have become undeniable; as Mia herself said at the start of my session with her, "I've already had like three meltdowns today."

Mia's emotional responses to her relationship with Dan are sending her a clear signal that she is not living a sexual life that is in line with her boundaries, wants, and needs or, at the very least, are flagging her down to pull over and assess the situation from the outside before continuing to speed down this sexual highway. Mia's experience is not uncommon and exists in a messy, human middle-ground in the context of the consent- and pleasure-based models of modern sexuality; as Mia tells me in her sessions, Dan never makes her feel unsafe, she likes their new relationship, she describes him as nice and caring, he asks for her consent, she gives it freely, and then she drives home and feels a mix of emotions including bad, sad, and anxious. If you asked Dan if he was practicing active consent with Mia, he would probably proudly say, "Yes!" and Mia would likely agree. However, it's clear from Mia's case that both could brush up on their sexual communication and consent skills, and for Mia, it's crucial that she knows and accepts herself and her own *yes*es, *no*s, and *maybe*s before she continues being sexual with Dan. This is where we return to erotic differentiation and to many of the strategies that have already been presented throughout this book.

Using This Book as a Guide toward Erotic Differentiation

A Step-by-Step Recap with Mia

It's clear that Mia's sexual ship needs to be righted, if not turned around entirely before more damage is done to the core development of her sexual self. Like so many people who come into my office looking for a compromise to solve their incompatible kinks, differing desire levels, and contradictory sexual tastes, Mia suffers from a lack of information about the options available for managing differences in an intimate partnership. And, like so many people hoping I'll serve them the perfect compromise on a silver platter, I disappoint by encouraging her to instead slowly back up and reestablish what is uniquely important to *her* before doing anything else. And, of course, I do this in the framework of erotic differentiation.

Erotic differentiation hinges on the continuous definition of the erotic self. This means that—surprise!—you've already been practicing erotic differentiation with the work contained within this book. So far, the preceding chapters have encouraged you to gain insight about and work on: 1) getting to know who you (really, actually) are as a complex sexual being, 2) sharing this sexual self-knowledge with your partner(s) in a way that is kind, clear, and easy to understand, and 3) asking them to share their own sexual selves with you, too. Guess what? All of this contributes to the greater goal of becoming better erotically differentiated and, happily, many of these skills can be gradually practiced with daily, simple actions. This means that as a therapist, I can encourage a client to move toward erotic differentiation without introducing it as a huge, complex topic, and that many erotically differentiated actions can be taken immediately.

Below is a step-by-step recap of how this book's chapters can guide us toward greater erotic differentiation and, more specifically, how the skills contained within them might be applied by Mia as she navigates her desire discrepancy with Dan in their brand-new relationship. Though these are organized in linear steps, these skills can be applied in whatever order feels right for you, and not all will apply to every single person's sexual conundrums. However you choose to use these skills is movement toward erotic differentiation and becoming a more authentic sexual person and partner.

Step 1: Acknowledge that the educational and social contexts in which we've been raised as sexual human beings are inherently flawed. Meaning: it's normal and natural to be unsure of how to do this whole sex thing. (See the Introduction and Chapter 1.)

For Mia: It doesn't make me "weird" or "abnormal" to be unsure of how to navigate sexual relationships, especially in a way that's honest and communication-forward. Actually, feeling unsure or like I haven't been adequately prepared for this makes me extremely normal and very much like the majority of my peers.

Step 2: Create your own image of what makes for good sex based on your own values, ideals, politics, and imagination. Pull from memories you have of good sex, or dream up what you want your future of good sex to look like, feel like, and include (return to worksheet "For Goodness Sex" in Chapter 1). Remember that ultimately, good sex is relational and hinges on your communication and relational skills.

For Mia: My vision of good sex includes an emotional connection before a physical, sexual connection. I want to have sexual experiences that easily accommodate a slower pace of "traditional progress" as imagined by my peers and have that feel unquestionably allowed.

Step 3: Sexual imposter syndrome is common (you're not alone!) and perfectly perfect sex isn't real (and that's good news!). Make goals for sex that are based on your authentic pleasure rather than on an ideal standard you've imagined or been told by peers, media, or porn. Failures may happen on your road to good sex and that's okay—trying and failing is how you get to know yourself and your partners, and how you get good at something! (See Chapter 2.)

For Mia: Plenty of people my age prefer to have sex later and at a slower progression. Prioritizing emotional connection before sexual connection may require me to have some slightly awkward conversations with dating app dates who might be expecting our sexual connection to happen faster because we met on an app.

Step 4: The Classic Mood is a barrier to authentically pleasurable sex and can be replaced by the Authentic Mood as long as you're willing to let it! Instead of prioritizing the mood, listen to your body, ask for what you want, and encourage all of your sexual partners to do the same, every time. (See Chapter 3.)

For Mia: Going with the flow of the Classic Mood with Dan so far has led me to move faster and violate my own boundaries in a way that isn't okay with me. I'm going to create an Authentic Mood by speaking up as soon as we are headed in a sexual direction that is beyond my boundaries.

Step 5: Identify your personal unhelpful automatic thoughts and Negative Narratives that are contributing to your unique Pleasure Pessimism that may be at play here. What do you believe about yourself and your own sexuality that is holding you back from creating a genuine sexual experience? Where did you learn the messages that contribute to these beliefs about yourself? What can you do to lessen their power over you and your sex life? (See Chapters 4 and 5.)

For Mia: I have thought that my "relative prudishness" must be the problem here and that the solution is to just get on with it and sexually catch up to Dan and my peers. I realize that this has been based on assumptions I've made from an outwardly sexualized atmosphere created among many of my peers and that it's okay for me to stand apart from that, to be different, and that I'm likely not the only person who feels this way, anyway. It's more important that I value myself more than I value what I think everyone else is doing.

Step 6: Dive into a Yes/ No/Maybe List to get in touch with what you really want, clarify what you don't want, and identify the sexual places you may be interested to explore, at the right time and with the right person/people. Not only is this a good exercise in self-defining your sexuality, it's excellent preparation for being able to communicate your boundaries and desires clearly and precisely to partners. (See Chapter 6.)

For Mia: A Yes/No/Maybe List helps me get clear about what I mean exactly by "a slower sexual pace." It helps me define certain sex acts, flavors of sex, and other sexual and relational pieces that feel exciting to me and those that do not. This better prepares me to communicate my wants and limits to Dan, and this list also helps me remember that, although I am currently highlighting a no *for myself and to Dan, I also have a lot of* yeses *that I want to include in my present-day sex life.*

Step 7: Ask for what you want from sex, from your partners, directly. This may feel risky for some valid reasons and for some historical, outdated reasons. Learn to better tell the difference between the two so you can know when to take the worthwhile risk of jumping into your authentic desires with *both* bravery *and* safety! Remember, rejection is protection, and asking is not demanding. (See Chapter 7.)

For Mia: I want to ask Dan to emotionally engage with me more so we can get to know each other outside of sex in a deeper way. I want to ask Dan to take a big step back from some of the specific sex acts we've been doing that have felt too fast. I worry that this will cause us to break up because I won't be sexually "enough" for him. If this does happen, I'll be okay and it will be good to have this incompatibility out in the open sooner rather than later. From what I know of Dan so far, I trust that he will respect my boundaries and hear me out.

Step 8: Set your sexual boundaries in order to better define your sexual desires and limits, even if this means that you may risk disappointing your partner(s). Have regular sexual feedback conversations with your ongoing sexual partner(s) as a way to continuously clarify your boundaries and collaborate on your best mutual sexual experiences. (See Chapter 8.)

For Mia: Being specific with Dan about things that felt good or didn't feel good in our past sexual experiences will be an important part of this shift in our sex life and will help me regularly check in with my own boundaries. This will also give Dan a better chance of getting to know who I actually am as a sexual person rather than just showing him a projection of what I think he wants. I hope to get to know more about him in this process, too.

Step 9: Prepare yourself to not only say *no*, but also to hear it! Do the groundwork on yourself to remove any misplaced triggers, internalized messages, or self-doubts that might emerge from someone sharing their boundaries with you or ultimately finding an incompatibility to be a dealbreaker. Learning to hear *no* like a pro (Chapter 9) is one important way to practice differentiation and to build your understanding of both yourself and your partner as unique sexual people with your own boundaries, needs, wants, and values. Remember that difference is not always the enemy to a fulfilling sex life. On the other hand, pretending that difference doesn't exist usually always is.

For Mia: It's possible that my clarity and boundaries around this will be a dealbreaker for Dan, who clearly is more comfortable with a faster pace of sex and is more sexually experienced than I am. I want to remind myself going forward that it's more important and ultimately more fulfilling and pleasurable for me to be having the sex I want to have, at the pace that helps me feel safe and comfortable, than it is for me to rush myself toward what I imagine to be Dan's wants and standards.

Mia did end up practicing erotic differentiation with Dan and found her happy ending. However, it didn't happen in the way most people would think a happy ending would. After laying all of their sexual cards out on Dan's plaid-printed sheets, Dan and Mia decided that yeah, they didn't feel sexually compatible enough to continue their sexual relationship after all. And this is good news for Mia, who left this situation with one of her fears confirmed yet survived (being rejected based on her sexual boundaries and lack of experience). Ultimately, she dodged what could have been a real sex-life–shaping catastrophe. In subsequent sessions, Mia and I discuss what she thinks might've happened if she and Dan had continued their sexual relationship in the direction it had been going before she started sexually self-defining. In all cases, what could have been between Mia and Dan, if she had continued to prioritize compromise, to protect the Classic Mood, and to imagine herself as the "broken one," doesn't look all that appealing to Mia (or, quite frankly, to me as her therapist). For those wondering if your relationship will always emerge out of this erotic differentiation approach intact, the answer is "No. But *you* will." And from an erotic differentiation standpoint, this—getting to deeply know and honor what is important to you *and* the other person—is exactly the point, not compromising to preserve the hologram of a forever-symbiotic relationship, even if it compromises you.

Though compromise might appear to solve sexual problems quickly, it rarely solves these problems authentically, honestly, or sustainably. The person who pushes down their desire for sex toys, kinks, or non-monogamy is likely to have that desire resurface, or it may even, what I call in therapy work, "come out sideways" through an affair, unhealthy porn compulsion, or other secretive or subconscious avenues. The person who assumes their "libido problem" is due to lack of exercise might never explore other possible causes, like unresolved relational strife or undesired sexual content (what I call *having the wrong kind of sex*). Or, as we can see in Mia's case, the more she pushed herself to have her sexual relationship with Dan develop at a faster rate than she wanted it too, the more shut down, disconnected, inauthentic, and distraught she became. If we instead approach common desire discrepancies from a place of erotic differentiation, the blaming of ourself and our partner(s) diminishes and longer-lasting, genuine solutions can present themselves, if and when they are available.

Though a solution that included the two of them continuing to date wasn't available to Mia and Dan, there are plenty of times when erotic differentiation presents solutions that keep partners together, like we saw with Brandon and Thom, Clark and Maria, Mark and Lisa, Jessa and Levi, and individual clients who practiced erotic differentiation in their casual dating lives like Kira, Jack, and Evan. And, now that Mia is more aware of her boundaries and more accepting of her desired pacing of sex, she can continue to date with these parameters in mind, so that she can find a match that's more suitable to her sexual style. When we keep a process of erotic differentiation at the forefront of our sex lives, we're more likely to bring authentic pleasure, self-valuing boundaries, genuine wants, and healthy curiosity about our partners along with it. Ultimately, this is the goal of my work with clients, as an educator, and of this book: to encourage people to live their sex lives with their honest desires, limits, and real human connection at the fore.

Maintaining a framework of erotic differentiation will be a trustworthy and productive North Star in your lifelong sexual journey if you let it. Knowing your sexual self deeply and being confident in your asks, desire-sharing, boundary setting, shame-shedding, and within all of your partner interactions (no matter how casual or committed) will keep all of your sexual experiences open to their fullest pleasure potential.

CONCLUSION

You're Doing It!

If I've written the sex advice book that I've set out to write, you'll be closing these chapters with a sexual to-do list longer than your favorite sex toy. Though the ultimate goal of my professional and personal work is to radically alter the way we are taught about, talk about, and experience sex, on an individual level, this kind of work is often granular. Sometimes this individual change happens intentionally (reading this book, working with a sex therapist, talking to your partner[s] about your boundaries) and sometimes it happens organically, sparked by a real-time catalyst (allowing yourself to have an explosive climax without worrying about what your face looks like, for example, and then feeling pleasurably inspired to never go back to the "old way" again). No matter how you set out to positively transform your sex life from here, the reality is that change has likely already happened, whether you're aware of it or not. Just by way of reading this book, you have shifted your relationship to your sex life, a small change that will lead to bigger changing if you allow yourself to stay open to it.

Though I spent the first chapters of this book disavowing the kind of one-and-done sex tips magazines love to advertise (advice pieces that, by the way, I have written plenty of myself), I do have one big, *real* sex secret to leave you with: authentically pleasurable sex cannot possibly exist unless you allow it to. In other words, learning how to talk about, think about, and actually have the sex you really, truly want starts with *you*.

Remember, you are a sexual person, not a sexual performance. The best sex ever is whatever the best sex ever is to you (and, when applicable, your partner[s]). Though this book has offered guiding maps of reframes, practices, questions, and strategies for creating your personal best sex life over time, giving yourself permission to have an authentically pleasurable sex life can happen right now, from wherever you are.

Who is your truest sexual self, actually? Cherish, protect, appreciate, celebrate, and maybe even have a big ol' orgasm with that person (you!) because without your truest sex self, there is no real pleasure to be had.

ACKNOWLEDGMENTS

As a 10-year-old I used to write and print a weekly newsletter for my family about relevant household news, like Mom's dish-washing strike or how my little sister had lost her hamster in the heating vents again (don't worry, he always turned up unscathed). I wrote and illustrated "books" about the afterlife adventures of our deceased family dog, short stories about getting my heart broken as a teenager, and once a long poem about my sister and the moon that won some kind of small-town award. On a few occasions, as a naive (perhaps future-telling) child, I told my mom that my life's goal was to be a "struggling writer." I loved writing and spent time doing it in some form nearly every day.

When I started my undergraduate program at Hampshire College, my intention was to major in creative writing, which quickly derailed toward a self-designed major in human sexuality after I took a class called "Youth, Sexuality & Education" in order to fulfill a social sciences requirement. Soon after, my career aspirations morphed into the predictable goal of being a sex columnist, what I saw as the perfect mash-up of my two interests.

It being the early 2000s I, of course, assumed that all sex writers' lives looked a lot like Carrie Bradshaw's, as depicted in HBO's *Sex and the City*. Once I was a sex columnist, I thought, I too would be draped in edgy, high fashion as I wrote "I couldn't help but wonder" theories about strangers' sex lives from the window of my New York City apartment, which I could somehow afford by doing only that and drinking whatever a cosmo was with my friends. Later in my young adulthood, I actually did get to be a sex columnist (still am!) and though it's a dream gig come true, it certainly isn't paying anyone's Manhattan rent. I adjusted my writing visions accordingly and, as a result, went to graduate school to become a therapist.

Still, I thought it rather exciting yet still very practical to assume that I'd eventually be writing my great sex-advice book while sipping espressos at one of my neighborhood's beautiful cafes, complete with the occasional trip to New York City to "do lunch with my agent."

Instead, I had just found out that I was pregnant with my son the very same week my soon-to-be agent contacted me with the opportunity to create a book proposal—an exciting surprise, followed by another exciting surprise, followed by a lot of angst about wanting to "have it all" and being terrified that I just logistically couldn't. Working full time as a therapist and baby-incubator, I slowly, slowly wrote the proposal throughout my pregnancy, maternity leave, and my son's world-rattling infancy (not advisable, by the way—I ended up throwing all of those sleep-deprived pages out).

But I did it! After all of the hard work to bring both a baby and a book proposal into the world, I victoriously signed my publishing contract in the spring of 2020—mere weeks after the COVID-19 pandemic hit the United States in earnest, and reality was setting in that our "two-week national quarantine" would in fact be much longer than that. My younger self never could've guessed that I would finally be writing my dream great-sex advice book during a worldwide, multi-year pandemic while quarantining at home with a toddler. And I couldn't help but wonder . . . was this a fucking joke?

Turns out my original fantasy experience of writing my book would be a lot less like a high-end fashion accessory and much more like a life-sustaining flotation device, something I clutched tightly as I—and everyone around me—was being tossed about in a tumultuous sea of unknowns, paradigm shifts, political unrest, racial violence, social-justice uprisings, crushing isolation, and, in our case, new parenting. By age 10, I knew that writing would always be my companion. But, I can truly say that before 2020, I had no idea that my relationship to writing would be quite like this.

Though much of 2020 happened in social distancing and isolation, the steadying practice of writing this book thankfully did not. The people who supported me in keeping this book—and, therefore, myself—afloat over the last three years have given me a thousand little gifts made of time, space, energy, motivation, encouragement, expertise, edits, and opportunity. Though I want to say thank you for every single one of these gifts, I've put a few down here.

First, thank you to all of the essential workers, health-care professionals, and scientists of modern medicine for bravely holding the frontlines of the COVID-19 crisis and for taking huge life risks in order to preserve ours. From delivering groceries to suiting up in garbage bags in order to treat COVID-19 patients, you will forever be the courageous, selfless heroes of my lifetime.

Thank you to my agent, Mary Krienke, for reading my writing in the first place and for liking it enough to reach out and remind me of my long-held, book-authoring dreams. Without your faith and enthusiasm, this little lifeboat of a book would have never left the dock.

Thank you to my editors, Rebecca Raskin and Emma Kupor, and the entire team at Harper Wave, for bringing this book to life. Rebecca, your personal investment in our shared vision for the future of sexuality made me sure from day one that this book would be in good hands. Thank you for cheering me on one chapter at a time, during a year when it was incredibly hard to muster up much cheer. Thank you, Emma, for bringing this project across the finish line at the final hour.

Thank you, Rebeca Soto, for your gorgeous illustrations and your similar commitment to a world full of consensual and genuine sexual pleasure and well-being. I'm so glad that this project included our collaboration, your passion, and your creative mind.

I'd like to rewind a little to say thank you to anyone who has ever published or edited my sex writing, especially Mark Roessler, who hired me as the *Valley Advocate*'s sex columnist over 10 years ago, an open door that I still credit for opening most others.

Thank you to the brick-and-mortar sex toy shops and the people who made them for taking me in, for lending me teaching space and floor models, and for teaching me more than anyone should know about dildos: Good Vibrations (San Francisco, CA), She Bop (Portland, OR), and especially Carol, Beth, and Constance of Oh My! Sensuality Shop in Northampton, MA.

Thank you to Rowe Senior High Camp campers, staff, and lifelong friends for showing me what an actual sex talk can and should look like. Your role modeling changed my life.

Thank you to my lifelong, deeply cherished friend Tenaya Schnare for every single thing you've done to shape my path, and especially for suggesting that I "talk about sex for a living" that one night when we were just 17 years old. That was a really good call.

Thank you to the many people who had a hand in teaching me how to be the kind of therapist I actually wanted to be: Emily, Brooke, Justine, Janet, CL, Donna, and Katherine (and, by extension, Ellyn Bader and Peter Pearson).

A long, continuous thank-you to the fellow, like-minded therapists I consider to be both close friends and the best professional consulting team I'll ever have: Hunter, Harlen, Knox, and especially Patrick, who has also doubled as a babysitter, dog sitter, and meme appreciator.

Thank you to my actual therapist, Julie, for 10-plus years of listening and support.

Thank you to the mentors, teachers, and role models in the various, intersecting fields of sex education, writing, and therapy who have inspired my work and have given me #goals to reach toward: Emily Nagoski, Esther Perel, Tristan Taormino, adrienne maree brown, and Carol Queen to name just a few.

Additionally, thank you to the people I consider to be my virtual colleagues in our pioneering field of independent sexuality professionals, some of whom I've never met in real life and may never meet at all. Your digital presence, advice, conversation, and support has taught me so much about this work and is something I have valued especially in these pandemic times: Erica Smith, Cameron Glover, Shaun Galanos, Lina Dune, Elle Stanger, Willow Howls, geunsaeng (olivia) ahn, Gabrielle Kassel, Elle Chase, Casia Sobolewski (previously Caitlin K. Roberts), Cassandra Corrado, Kai Werder, Sophia Wallace, Luna Matatas, Allison Moon, Goddess Cecilia Villero, Robyn Manning-Samuels, Mia Little, Cory Bush, Lauren Hamilton-Soulé, Andre Shakti, and Jiz Lee. Thank you for all of the reposts, repping, and rooting me on—I consider myself very lucky to work alongside all of you.

To my clients and sex column write-ins, thank you for trusting me with your sex lives, relationships, trauma, healing, and stories. Your vulnerability, strength, humor, bravery, and ability to change your patterns within oppressive sex educational systems impresses me endlessly. I'm grateful to witness your evolutions and am honored to be part of your process.

Thank you to my inner-circle folks who have nourished me with food, affection, listening ears, and never-ending text threads: Lex, Gabe, Ian, Laura, Rinat, Kyla, Jes, Ron, Tavish, Shane, Ember, David, Ruby, and Elena (who also gets an extra thank-you for taking such good care of Rocko).

A long thank-you across time zones to Lily Brooks-Dalton for everything, really. You've been an invaluable anchor, consultant, and unbeatable force of friendship in my life, 3,000 miles of states be damned.

Thank you to those who will remain anonymous that have been a part of my real-life, experiential sex education and self-discovery (with a special thank-you to those of you who gave me your blessings to print my version of our stories). Many of you have held me in my most vulnerable human moments, and I don't take that gift for granted.

Thank you to (all of) my parents, who have always supported my nontraditional professional aspirations, even if doing so meant reading (perhaps skimming?) some stories about your daughter that, in normal circumstances, you would probably really rather not. Thank you especially to my sister, Rory, for being my confidant, hilarious laugh twin, and sometimes worthy opponent since I was just four years old—I love you so much.

Thank you to Grammy for giving our new family some of its most valuable support in the form of weekly childcare, schedule upkeep, and helping us raise the best little guy I know.

The most intimate kind of gratitude goes to my co-parent, Wyatt, for jumping into the deep end of the unknown with me and doing so with hope, joy, and abandon. If Pleasure Optimism were a way of life, you'd be it.

And finally, thank you to my toddler, Rocko, for being the brightest star my galaxy has ever seen just by way of being yourself. May the landscape of sex education change so positively in the next 15 years that you never feel compelled to read this book yourself. But, if you do decide to read it, just pretend that your own mother didn't write it because, hey, the information's probably still good.

RESOURCE GUIDE

This guide is a small sampling of what's available in the big, ever-expanding world of sexuality resources, educators, and websites. Studies show that choice overload—our decreasing ability to make a satisfying choice between several options—kicks in somewhere after having six to 12 items to choose from. So, in each category below, that is about how many options you'll find. Of course, this means many great options may be missing, and I hope that by way of exploring the options listed below, you'll find even more exciting resources yourself.

Here in this guide you'll find all kinds of sex and sexuality resources in the form of books, websites, conferences, and sometimes individual educators themselves who create great educational content on their websites or social media accounts. Note that some of this information may have become outdated in the time it took this book to make it into your hands, but either way, this resource guide should provide you with a good start to your continued pleasure-based sex education. Happy learning!

Sexual Pleasure and Adult Sex Ed
- *Pleasure Activism* by adrienne maree brown
- *Come as You Are* by Emily Nagoski
- *Carnal Knowledge* by Zoë Ligon
- *The Secrets of Great G-Spot Orgasms and Female Ejaculation* by Tristan Taormino

- *Curvy Girl Sex* by Elle Chase
- *What Fresh Hell Is This?: Perimenopause, Menopause, Other Indignities, and You* by Heather Corinna
- *The Ultimate Guide to Sex and Disability* by Miriam Kaufman, Cory Silverberg, and Fran Odette
- Oh Joy Sex Toy: a sex education and toy review comic, ohjoysextoy.com
- Afrosexology: webinars, workshops, and resources, afrosexology.com/links
- Sexual Health Includes Pleasure (SHIP), Providence, Rhode Island: Virtual adult sex education and pleasure workshops, weknowship.org
- Dawn Serra's Explore More Summit, exploremoresummit.com
- The S.L.A.M. (Sexuality Liberators and Movers) Conference, stephaniespeakshere.com/s-l-a-m
- Bethany Gehman with the Deaf Sexual Wellness Center, linktr.ee/jooux or on Instagram @joouxcenter
- The Cliteracy Project by Sophia Wallace, sophiawallace.art

Sexual and Relational Communication
- *Tongue Tied* by Stella Harris
- *Unf*ck Your Boundaries* by Faith G. Harper
- *Unf*ck Your Intimacy* by Faith G. Harper
- *What to Say Next: Successful Communication in Work, Life, and Love—with Autism Spectrum Disorder* by Sarah Nannery and Larry Nannery

Anal Sex
- *Anal Sex Basics* by Carlyle Jansen
- *The Ultimate Guide to Prostate Pleasure* by Charlie Glickman and Aislinn Emirzian
- *The Ultimate Guide to Anal Sex for Women* by Tristan Taormino
- *Anal Pleasure and Health* by Jack Morin

Queer Sex and Sexuality
(Note: Many of the other resources listed in this guide are queer-inclusive.)

- *Girl Sex 101* by Allison Moon
- *Queer Sex: A Trans and Non-Binary Guide to Intimacy, Pleasure, and Relationships* by Juno Roche
- *Bliss Club: Sex Tips for Creative Lovers* by Jüne Plã
- *The Whole Lesbian Sex Book* by Felice Newman
- *The Trans Partner Handbook: A Guide for When Your Partner Transitions* by Jo Green
- *Pronouns: A Resource* on GLSEN.org
- *Trans* Ally Workbook* by Davey Shlasko

Masturbation and Solo Sex
- *Bang!: Masturbation for People of All Genders and Abilities* by Vic Liu
- *The Ultimate Guide to Solo Sex* by Jenny Block
- *Getting Off* by Jamye Waxman
- *Sex for One* by Betty Dodson

Porn and Erotica
(Mostly feminist, ethically made, women-centric, and queer options)
- AORTA Films, aortafilms.com
- Pink and White Productions, pinklabel.tv
- The Feminist Porn Awards, feministpornawards.com
- Make Love Not Porn, makelovenotporn.tv
- Lady Cheeky, ellechase.com/ladycheeky
- Dipsea: Sexy audio stories, dipseastories.com
- Spit, spit.exposed
- Jet Setting Jasmine and King Noire, jsjlinks.com or Instagram @jetsetjasmine and @therealkingnoire
- Cleis Press: Publisher of erotica anthologies and sex educational guides, cleispress.com

Kink and BDSM (Bondage and Dominance/Dominance and Submission/Sadism and Masochism)
- *The Ultimate Guide to Kink* by Tristan Taormino
- *The New Topping Book* by Dossie Easton and Janet W. Hardy

- *The New Bottoming Book* by Dossie Easton and Janet W. Hardy
- *Showing You the Ropes* by the Two Knotty Boys
- *The Seductive Art of Japanese Bondage* by Midori
- Shibari Study, Instagram @shibari.study, shibaristudy.com
- Lina Dune: BDSM and kink content creator and educator, Instagram @askasub, patreon.com/askasub

Non-Monogamy, Polyamory, and Open Relationships

- *Opening Up* by Tristan Taormino
- *More Than Two* by Eve Rickert and Franklin Veaux
- *The Ethical Slut* by Janet W. Hardy and Dossie Easton
- *Love's Not Color Blind* by Kevin A. Patterson
- *Polysecure: Attachment, Trauma, and Consensual Non-Monogamy* by Jessica Fern
- *The Jealousy Workbook: Exercises and Insights for Managing Open Relationships* by Kathy Labriola
- *Sex at Dawn* by Christopher Ryan and Cacilda Jethá

Relationships, Therapy, and Problem-Solving

- *It Takes One to Tango* by Winifred M. Reilly
- *The State of Affairs* by Esther Perel
- *Mating in Captivity* by Esther Perel
- *Daring Greatly* by Brené Brown
- *The New Rules of Marriage* by Terrence Real
- *In Quest of the Mythical Mate* by Ellyn Bader and Peter Pearson
- *Wired for Love* by Stan Tatkin
- *Attached* by Amir Levine and Rachel Heller
- Shaun Galanos: Love Coach and Educator, teaches many digital courses on love and relationships, shaungalanos.com/hello or Instagram @thelovedrive

Sex Ed and Consent for Kids, Teens, and Parents

- *Wait, What? A Comic Book Guide to Relationships, Bodies, and Growing Up* by Heather Corinna, Isabella Rotman, and Luke Howard
- *Let's Talk about It: The Teen's Guide to Sex, Relationships, and Being a Human* by Erika Moen and Matthew Nolan

- *The Every Body Book: The LGBTQ+ Inclusive Guide for Kids about Sex, Gender, Bodies, and Families* by Rachel E. Simon
- *Sex Is a Funny Word* by Cory Silverberg and Fiona Smyth
- Scarleteen: Sex Ed for the Real World, scarleteen.com
- Sex Positive Families, LLC, bio.fm/sexpositivefamilies, Instagram @sexpositive_families
- Dr. Nadine Thornhill: Certified sex educator and EdD specializing in child and adolescent sexuality, nadinethornhill.com, Instagram @nadinethornhill
- *The Ultimate Guide to Sex through Pregnancy and Motherhood* by Madison Young
- *Boys & Sex* by Peggy Orenstein
- *Girls & Sex* by Peggy Orenstein

Sex, Sexuality, and Disability

- *The Ultimate Guide to Sex and Disability* by Miriam Kaufman, Cory Silverberg, and Fran Odette
- *A Quick & Easy Guide to Sex & Disability* by A. Andrews
- *BANG!: Masturbation for People of All Genders and Abilities* by Vic Liu
- The Disability and Sexuality Access Network (DASANetwork), dasanetwork.org
- Andrew Gurza: Disability awareness consultant and podcaster on *Disability After Dark*, Instagram @andrewgurza_, patreon.com/disabilityafterdark
- Alex Dacy: Disability representation and body confidence blogger and creator, Instagram @wheelchair_rapunzel
- Bethany Gehman with the Deaf Sexual Wellness Center, linktr.ee/jooux or on Instagram @joouxcenter

Relationship Safety, Abuse, and Survivorship

- *Healing Sex* by Staci Haines
- *The Sexual Healing Journey* by Wendy Maltz
- *Invitations to Responsibility: The Therapeutic Engagement of Men Who Are Violent and Abusive* by Alan Jenkins
- *Victims No Longer: The Classic Guide for Men Recovering from Sexual Child Abuse* by Mike Lew

- *The Courage to Heal: A Guide for Women Survivors of Child Sexual Abuse* by Ellen Bass and Lauren Davis
- "The Abuse Checklist," https://www.scarleteen.com/bb/viewtopic.php?f=16&t=20
- The Transgender Sexual Violence Project by FORGE, forge-forward.org
- National Coalition of Anti-Violence Programs: National Advocacy for Local LGBTQ Communities, avp.org

Callouts, Call-Ins, Canceling, and Conflict Resolution

- *We Will Not Cancel Us: And Other Dreams of Transformative Justice* by adrienne maree brown
- *Accountability in Restorative Justice* by Declan Roche
- "Why Demonizing Call-Out Culture Perpetuates Racism" by Katrice Dustin published on i-d.vice.com
- "Calling In vs. Calling Out: How to Talk about Inclusion" by Maya Hu-Chan published on Inc.com
- "Reframing Cancel Culture: Why Calling Someone Out Is an Act of Service" by Erin Bunch published on wellandgood.com
- "9 Ways to Be Accountable When You've Been Abusive" by Kai Cheng Thom published on everydayfeminism.com
- Arise Embodiment: Trauma-informed conflict resolution services and resources by Kai Cheng Thom, ariseembodiment.org

Small Businesses to Shop With

Sex Toys and Accessories
- Unbound, unboundbabes.com
- Shop Enby, shopenby.com
- Honey Play Box, honeyplaybox.com
- She Bop (Portland, OR), sheboptheshop.com
- Oh My! Sensuality Shop (Northampton, MA)
- Dynamo (New Orleans, LA), shop.dynamotoys.com
- Feelmore (Oakland, CA), feelmore510.com

- Awakening Boutique (Denver, CO), awakeningboutique.com
- As You Like It (Eugene, OR), asyoulikeitshop.com
- Spectrum Boutique (Detroit, MI), spectrumboutique.com

Kink and Leather Gear
- Mr. S Leather (San Francisco, CA), mr-s-leather.com
- Leather Coven (Holyoke, MA), leathercoven.etsy.com or Instagram @leathercoven
- H.O.S. Leather, hosleather.com or Instagram @hos_leather
- Rand Leather (Atlanta, GA), randleather.com or Instagram @randleather
- Kolby Brianne Leather, kolbybrianne.com or Instagram @kolbybrianneleather
- Gnat Glitter Kink, gnat.shop or Instagram @gnat_glitter_kink

Sex Work and Sex Workers Resources

- *Coming Out Like a Porn Star: Essays on Pornography, Protection, and Privacy* edited by Jiz Lee
- *Thriving in Sex Work: Heartfelt Advice for Staying Sane in the Sex Industry* by Lola Davina
- *Revolting Prostitutes: The Fight for Sex Workers' Rights* by Juno Mac and Molly Smith
- *Playing the Whore: The Work of Sex Work* by Melissa Gira Grant
- Sex Workers Outreach Project: A national social justice network dedicated to the fundamental human rights of people involved in the sex trade, swopusa.org

Becoming a Sex Educator or Sexuality Professional
- *Becoming a Sexuality Professional: A Beginner's Guide to Finding Their Way within Sex Ed* (eBook) by Cameron Glover, www.successfulsexed.com
- Successful Sex Ed: Premium professional development for sexuality professionals, www.successfulsexed.com

- Black Sweat: A professional development opportunity to learn from emergent and seasoned Black sexuality professionals, anteuppd.com
- *Black and Sexy: A Framework of Racialized Sexuality* by Tracie Q. Gilbert
- "Sex Educator Starter Kit" (pre-recorded webinar, 2019), yanatallonhicks.com/sexedstarterkit
- "Consent & Cookies: A Pre-recorded Webinar for Sex Educators, Teachers, and Facilitators," yanatallonhicks.com/recorded -consent-webinar
- Tristan Taormino's Sex Educator Boot Camp, sexeducatorbootcamp .com
- Institute for Sexuality and Enlightenment (ISEE): Holistic sex education training for clinicians and educators, instituteforsexuality .com
- Sex Down South: Atlanta Sexuality Conference, sexdownsouth.com
- American Association of Sexuality Educators, Counselors, and Therapists (AASECT), aasect.org

NOTES

A Couple of Brief Notes

1   by way of white privilege: Fleming, Crystal. *How to Be Less Stupid about Race: On Racism, White Supremacy, and the Racial Divide.* Boston: Beacon Press, 2019.

2   past and current: Morris, Amanda. "'You Just Feel Like Nothing': California to Pay Sterilization Victims." *New York Times*, July 11, 2021.

3   racist reproductive health research practices: Roberts, Dorothy E. *Killing the Black Body: Race, Reproduction, and the Meaning of Liberty.* New York: Vintage, 2017.

Introduction: Hey! We're All Getting Screwed! (by Sex Education)

1   to 500 strangers: Tallon-Hicks, Yana. "Is the Porn Brain Our New Sex Educator?" TEDxViennaSalon, May 18, 2016. YouTube video. https://www.youtube.com/watch?v=lxlGFtg4Z2c.

2   modern Our Whole Lives (O.W.L.) programs: Sprung, Barbara, Dawn Casey, and Tom Goldsmith. "Our Whole Lives: Lifespan Sexuality Education." Unitarian Universalist Association, retrieved January 11, 2021. https://www.uua.org/re/owl.

3   medically accurate information: Eisenstein, Zach. "Lack of State Sex Ed Regulation Puts Students in Danger of Receiving Harmful Lessons, Report Finds" SIECUS, March 5, 2020. https://siecus.org/state-profiles-2019-announcement.

4   preferred option for safer sex: Eisenstein, Zach. "Lack of State Sex Ed Regulation Puts Students in Danger of Receiving Harmful Lessons, Report Finds" SIECUS, March 5, 2020. https://siecus.org/state-profiles-2019-announcement/.

5 of all industrialized countries: "Adolescent Pregnancy and Its Outcomes Across Countries." Guttmacher Institute, August 2015. https://www.guttmacher.org/fact-sheet/adolescent-pregnancy-and -its-outcomes-across-countries.

6 25 European countries: Ketting, Evert, and Olena Ivanova. "Sexuality Education in Europe and Central Asia." International Planned Parenthood Federation, 2016. https://www.euro.who.int/__data/assets/pdf_file /0010/379054/BZgA_IPPFEN_ComprehensiveStudyReport_Online.pdf.

7 more often than their U.S. counterparts: Currie, Candace, Cara Zanotti, Anthony Morgan, et al. Rep. *Social Determinants of Health and Well-Being among Young People*. Copenhagen: WHO Regional Office for Europe, 2012.

8 lowest teen pregnancy rates: The World Bank. "Adolescent Fertility Rate (Births per 1,000 Women Ages 15–19)." Adolescent Fertility Rate, 2019. https://data.worldbank.org/indicator/SP.ADO.TFRT.

9 at an earlier age: Currie, Candace, Cara Zanotti, Anthony Morgan, et al. Rep. *Social Determinants of Health and Well-Being among Young People*. Copenhagen: WHO Regional Office for Europe, 2012.

10 first sexual experiences: de Melker, Saskia. "The Case for Starting Sex Education in Kindergarten." *PBS NewsHour*, May 27, 2015. https://www.pbs.org/newshour/health/spring-fever.

11 a booming #MeToo movement: #MeToo Movement, retrieved April 14, 2021. https://metoomvmt.org.

12 just don't have: Kosciw, Joseph, Emily Greytak, Neal Palmer, and Madelyn Boesen. "The 2013 National School Climate Survey." The Gay, Lesbian, & Straight Education Network, 2014. https://www .glsen.org/research/2013-national-school-climate-survey.

13 60 percent of girls: Sabina, Chiara, Janis Wolak, and David Finkelhor. "The Nature and Dynamics of Internet Pornography Exposure for Youth." *CyberPsychology & Behavior* 11, no. 6 (2008): 691–93. https://doi.org/10.1089/cpb.2007.0179.

14 intentionally sought out porn: Rothman, Emily F., Courtney Kaczmarsky, Nina Burke, Emily Jansen, and Allyson Baughman. "'Without Porn . . . I Wouldn't Know Half the Things I Know Now': A Qualitative Study of Pornography Use among a Sample of Urban, Low-Income, Black and Hispanic Youth." *Journal of Sex Research* 52, no. 7 (2014): 736–46. https:// doi.org/10.1080/00224499.2014.960908.

15 nine years old: Rothman, Emily F., Courtney Kaczmarsky, Nina Burke, Emily Jansen, and Allyson Baughman. "'Without Porn . . . I Wouldn't Know Half the Things I Know Now': A Qualitative Study of Pornography Use Among a Sample of Urban, Low-Income, Black and Hispanic Youth." *Journal of Sex Research* 52, no. 7 (2014): 736–46. https://doi.org/10.1080/00224499.2014.960908.

16 "virginity loss": Although this statistic is worded as "virginity loss," virginity is a complex social construct that typically defines "virginity" as a person's first experience with penis-in-vagina penetration. This fails to take into account varieties of sexuality, gender, sex acts, and what might constitute an individual experience of virginity. I prefer the term "sexual debut," which is more inclusively defined as a person's self-determined first sexual experience, however they choose to define said sexual experience for themselves.

17 17 years old: "Key Statistics from the National Survey of Family Growth- S Listing." Centers for Disease Control and Prevention, August 14, 2017. https://www.cdc.gov/nchs/nsfg/key_statistics/s.htm.

18 accurate sex education: Jones, Maggie. "What Teenagers Are Learning from Online Porn." *New York Times Magazine*, February 7, 2018. https://www.nytimes.com/2018/02/07/magazine/teenagers-learning -online-porn-literacy-sex-education.html.

19 one Boston University study: Rothman, Emily F., Courtney Kaczmarsky, Nina Burke, Emily Jansen, and Allyson Baughman. "'Without Porn . . . I Wouldn't Know Half the Things I Know Now': A Qualitative Study of Pornography Use Among a Sample of Urban, Low-Income, Black and Hispanic Youth." *The Journal of Sex Research* 52, no. 7 (2014): 736–46. https://doi.org/10.1080/00224499.2014.960908.

20 in order to climax: Marin, Vanessa. "How to Stop Worrying about How Long It Takes You to Orgasm." *Bustle*, October 24, 2019. https:// www.bustle.com/wellness/how-long-should-it-take-a-woman-to -come-how-to-stop-worrying-during-sex-3797099.

Chapter 1: On Good (Sexual) Relations

1 "that is broken": Nagoski, Emily. *Come as You Are: The Surprising New Science That Will Transform Your Sex Life*. New York: Simon & Schuster, 2015.

2 awkward sexual moments: Though, pulling sudden moves like these with someone certainly could violate their consent but we'll get into that later in Chapter 10.

3 merit-based competition: Dunbar-Ortiz, Roxanne. *An Indigenous Peoples' History of the United States*. Boston: Beacon Press, 2014.

4 out of the conversation: Eisenstein, Zach. "Lack of State Sex Ed Regulation Puts Students in Danger of Receiving Harmful Lessons, Report Find" SIECUS, March 5, 2020. https://siecus.org/state-profiles-2019-announcement.

5 your partner first: Rehman, Uzma S., Alessandra H. Rellini, and Erin Fallis. "The Importance of Sexual Self-Disclosure to Sexual Satisfaction and Functioning in Committed Relationships." *Journal of Sexual Medicine* 8, no. 11 (2011): P3108–3115. https://doi.org/10.1111/j.1743-6109.2011.02439.x.

6 more fulfilling sex: Montesi, Jennifer L., Bradley T. Conner, Elizabeth A. Gordon, Robert L. Fauber, Kevin H. Kim, and Richard G. Heimberg. "On the Relationship among Social Anxiety, Intimacy, Sexual Communication, and Sexual Satisfaction in Young Couples." *Archives of Sexual Behavior* 42, no. 1 (2013): 81–91. https://doi.org/10.1007/s10508-012-9929-3.

7 ethical and legal sex: Sex without consent can be understood as rape and not actually as sex at all. This is because *sex* is colloquially understood as a shared sexual experience between parties, which can *only* occur when consent is present.

8 key physiological components: Nagoski, Emily. *Come as You Are: The Surprising New Science That Will Transform Your Sex Life*. New York: Simon & Schuster, 2015.

9 restorative justice process: Though diving into the complex topics of accountability and restorative justice is beyond the scope of this book, they are relevant companion topics that you can look into via the published experts in their field. See the resource guide for a few suggestions to get you started.

10 restorative justice process: Roche, Declan. *Accountability in Restorative Justice*. Oxford, England: Oxford University Press, 2003.

11 a subjectively satisfying sex life: Johnson, Susan. "Why Emotional Safety Is the Defining Feature of Good Sex." Psychotherapy

Networker, 2016. https://www.psychotherapynetworker.org/blog /details/783/why-emotional-safety-is-the-defining-feature-of-good.

12 open communication: Khoury, Clautilde B., and Bruce M. Findlay. "What Makes for Good Sex? The Associations among Attachment Style, Inhibited Communication and Sexual Satisfaction." *Journal of Relationships Research* 5 (2014). https://doi.org/10.1017/jrr.2014.7.

13 links shame and silence together: Brown, Brené. "Listening to Shame." *TED, March 2012.* https://www.ted.com/talks/brene_brown_listening _to_shame.

14 lack of communication: Byers, E. Sandra. "Beyond the *Birds and the Bees* and *Was It Good for You?*: Thirty Years of Research on Sexual Communication." *Canadian Psychology/Psychologie canadienne* 52, no. 1 (2011): 20–8. https://doi.org/10.1037/a0022048.

15 automatic thoughts: Automatic thoughts are instantaneous, habitual, and nonconscious ways of thinking about ourselves, our situations, and the people around us. In the field of psychology, automatic thoughts are understood to affect a person's mood and actions. More on automatic thoughts and your sex life in Chapter 5.

16 with your consent: Psst, don't despair, these responses can be really hard work in some circumstances, so there's an entire chapter devoted to just this, Chapter 9: How to Hear *No* Like a Pro.

Chapter 2: Your Perfectly Imperfect Sex Life

1 "I feel alive": Lahiri, Jhumpa. *In Other Words.* London: Vintage Books, 2017.

2 Seventy percent of people: Young, Valerie. *The Secret Thoughts of Successful Women: Why Capable People Suffer from the Impostor Syndrome and How to Thrive in Spite of It.* New York: Crown Business, 2011.

3 even Neil Armstrong: Gaiman, Neil. "The Neil Story (with Additional Footnote)." Neil Gaiman's Journal, May 17, 2017. https://journal .neilgaiman.com/2017/05/the-neil-story-with-additional-footnote. html.

4 systemic oppressions: McGee, Ebony O., Portia K. Botchway, Dara E. Naphan-Kingery, Amanda J. Brockman, Stacey Houston II, and Devin T. White. "Racism Camouflaged as Impostorism and the Im-

pact on Black STEM Doctoral Students." *Race Ethnicity and Education* (2021): 1–21. https://doi.org/10.1080/13613324.2021.1924137.

5 in mainstream porn and media: Byron, Paul, Alan McKee, Ash Watson, Katerina Litsou, and Roger Ingham. "Reading for Realness: Porn Literacies, Digital Media, and Young People." *Sexuality & Culture* 25 (2021): 786–805. https://doi.org/10.1007/s12119-020-09794-6.

6 researchers and psychologists recommend: Young, Valerie. *The Secret Thoughts of Successful Women: Why Capable People Suffer from the Impostor Syndrome and How to Thrive in Spite of It.* New York: Crown Business, 2011.

7 or numbing out: Donahue, John J. "Fight-Flight-Freeze System." *Encyclopedia of Personality and Individual Differences* (2020): 1590–95. https://doi.org/10.1007/978-3-319-24612-3_751.

8 her excellent book *Come as You Are*: Nagoski, Emily. *Come as You Are: The Surprising New Science That Will Transform Your Sex Life.* New York: Simon & Schuster, 2015.

9 traditional imposter syndrome: Bravata, Dena, Divya Madhusudhan, Michael Boroff, and Kevin Cokley. "Commentary: Prevalence, Predictors, and Treatment of Imposter Syndrome: A Systematic Review." *Journal of Mental Health & Clinical Psychology* 4, no. 3 (2020): 12–16. https://doi.org/10.29245/2578-2959/2020/3.1207.

10 in a fixed mindset: A fixed mindset refers to people who see their qualities (or, in this context, their sexuality or sexual ability) as fixed traits that cannot change.

11 cognitive behavioral therapy (CBT): Beck, Judith S. *Cognitive Behavior Therapy: Basics and Beyond*, 3rd edition. New York: Guilford Press, 2020.

12 many evidence-based studies: Tolin, David F. "Is Cognitive–Behavioral Therapy More Effective than Other Therapies?: A Meta-Analytic Review." *Clinical Psychology Review* 30, no. 6 (2010): 710–20. https://doi.org/10.1016/j.cpr.2010.05.003.

13 the research on resilient people: Helmreich, Isabella, Angela Kunzler, Andrea Chmitorz, Jochem König, Harald Binder, Michèle Wessa, and Klaus Lieb. "Psychological Interventions for Resilience Enhancement in Adults." *Cochrane Database of Systematic Reviews* (2017). https://doi.org/10.1002/14651858.cd012527.

14 "pleasure is the measure": Nagoski, Emily. *Come as You Are: The Surprising New Science That Will Transform Your Sex Life*. New York: Simon & Schuster, 2015.

Chapter 3: Barrier #1: The Mood

1 "leads us to self-knowledge": Walker, Alice. "Book Shows Lessons from Ancient People." Interview with Miles O'Brien. CNN.com, October 12, 1998. http://edition.cnn.com/books/dialogue/9810/alice.walker.

2 *The Good Vibrations Guide to the G-Spot:* Winks, Cathy. *The Good Vibrations Guide: The G-Spot*. San Francisco: Down There Press, 1998.

3 German physician Ernst Gräfenberg: Gräfenberg, Ernst. "The Role of Urethra in Female Orgasm." *International Journal of Sexology* 3, no. 3 (1950): 145–48.

4 sex-negative study: Salama, Samuel, Florence Boitrelle, Amélie Gauquelin, Lydia Malagrida, Nicolas Thiounn, and Pierre Desvaux. "Nature and Origin of 'Squirting' in Female Sexuality." *Journal of Sexual Medicine* 12, no. 3 (2015): 661–66. https://doi.org/10.1111/jsm.12799.

5 My sex column: Tallon-Hicks, Yana. "Yanatallonhicks.com." Retrieved June 11, 2020. https://yanatallonhicks.com/blog.

6 *The Good Vibrations Guide to the G Spot:* Winks, Cathy. *The Good Vibrations Guide: The G-Spot* . San Francisco: Down There Press, 1998.

7 at heyepiphora.com: Hey Epiphora. "My Love, the Pure Wand (+ a Few Tips)." *Hey Epiphora* (blog), July 26, 2010. https://heyepiphora.com/my-love-the-pure-wand-plus-a-few-tips.

8 by Tristan Taormino: Taormino, Tristan. *The Secrets of Great G-Spot Orgasms and Female Ejaculation: The Best Positions and Latest Techniques for Creating Powerful, Long-Lasting Full-Body Orgasms*. Beverly, MA: Quiver, 2011.

Chapter 4: Barrier #2: Pleasure Pessimism

1 "that created it": Hawley, Pamela. "Einstein Said It: 'No Problem Can Be Solved from the Same Level of Consciousness That Created It.'" Living and Giving, May 16, 2016. https://pamelahawley.wordpress.com/2016/05/16/einstein-said-it-no-problem-can-be-solved-from-the-same-consciousness-that-created-it.

2   "can't have nice things": "This Is Why We Can't Have Nice Things." Wiktionary, last edited March 31, 2021. https://en.wiktionary.org/wiki/this_is_why_we_can%27t_have_nice_things.

3   in order to climax: Bhat, Gajanan S., and Anuradha Shastry. "Time to Orgasm in Women in a Monogamous Stable Heterosexual Relationship." *Journal of Sexual Medicine* 17, no. 4 (2020): 749–60. https://doi.org/10.1016/j.jsxm.2020.01.005.

4   solely from sexual intercourse: Wallen, Kim, and Elisabeth A. Lloyd. "Female Sexual Arousal: Genital Anatomy and Orgasm in Intercourse." *Hormones and Behavior* 59, no. 5 (2011): 780–92. https://doi.org/10.1016/j.yhbeh.2010.12.004.

5   your sexual desires or habits: Automatic thoughts and beliefs about our consensual sex lives are different than flashbacks, triggered reactions, or other responses to trauma that may occur during sex, if you are someone with a history of trauma. Therefore, the treatment or approach to said thoughts should be handled differently and with more deliberate caution and expertise than the suggestions that are made in this chapter. If you would like more information or help in working through trauma responses during sex, please see the resource guide.

6   Cognitive Behavioral Therapy (CBT): Beck, Judith S. *Cognitive Behavior Therapy: Basics and Beyond, 3rd edition*. New York: Guilford Press, 2020.

7   anxiety, depression, and phobias: Twomey, C., G. O'Reilly, and M. Byrne. "Effectiveness of Cognitive Behavioural Therapy for Anxiety and Depression in Primary Care: A Meta-Analysis." *European Psychiatry* 30 (2015): 261. https://doi.org/10.1016/s0924-9338(15)31860-5; McAleavey, Andrew A., Louis G. Castonguay, and Marvin R. Goldfried. "Clinical Experiences in Conducting Cognitive-Behavioral Therapy for Social Phobia." *Behavior Therapy* 45, no. 1 (2014): 21–35. https://doi.org/10.1016/j.beth.2013.09.008.

8   the research behind CBT: Beck, Judith S. *Cognitive Behavior Therapy: Basics and Beyond, 3rd edition*. New York: Guilford Press, 2020.

9   *secondary gains*: van Egmond, J. J. "Multiple Meanings of Secondary Gain." *American Journal of Psychoanalysis* 63, no. 2 (2003): 135–47.

Chapter 5: Reshaping Negative Narratives

1 "the good ones": Roger, Jodie. "The Stories We Tell Ourselves." TEDxBerkleeValencia, August 27, 2014. YouTube video. https://www.youtube.com/watch?v=PXxBRhYseNY.

2 extremely common: Pastuszak, Alexander W. "Current Diagnosis and Management of Erectile Dysfunction." *Current Sexual Health Reports* 6, no. 3 (2014): 164–76. https://doi.org/10.1007/s11930-014 -0023-9.

3 *Negative Narratives*: Agas, Jessica. "The Effect of Narrative on Health." *3808: A Journal of Critical Writing* 10 (2015): 61–5.

4 "brave five minutes longer": Eastman, Fred. *Playing Square with Tomorrow*. New York: Published jointly by Council of Women for home missions and Missionary Education Movement, 1921.

5 "brave five minutes longer": I've slightly edited this quote for gender inclusivity.

6 serious medical conditions: Wyllie, Michael G. "The Underlying Pathophysiology and Causes of Erectile Dysfunction." *Clinical Cornerstone* 7, no. 1 (2005): 19–26. https://doi.org/10.1016/s1098 -3597(05)80045-6.

7 doesn't flawlessly correlate: Nagoski, Emily. *Come as You Are: The Surprising New Science That Will Transform Your Sex Life*. New York: Simon & Schuster, 2015

Chapter 6: How to Discover What You Want

1 same old sex routine: Perel, Esther. *Mating in Captivity: Reconciling the Erotic and the Domestic*. New York: HarperCollins, 2009.

2 The Yes/No/Maybe List: Osworth, A. E. "You Need Help: Here Is a Worksheet to Help You Talk to Partners about Sex." Autostraddle, June 19, 2014. https://www.autostraddle.com/you-need-help-here -is-a-worksheet-to-help-you-talk-to-partners-about-sex-237385; Corinna, Heather, and CJ Turett. "Yes, No, Maybe So: A Sexual Inventory Stocklist." Scarleteen, updated July 10, 2019. https://www.scarleteen.com/article/advice/yes_no_maybe_so_a_sexual _inventory_stocklist.

3 McCloud, RC "Yes or No or Maybe." That Other Paper, March 22, 2007. http://www.thatotherpaper.com/austin/yes_no_maybe.

4 Non-monogamous: For extensive information on consensual non-monogamy and the various non-monogamous relationship structures listed on page 199 refer to the resource guide.

5 Aftercare: Fuentes, Sage. "Caring about Aftercare: Thesis Presentation of Initial Findings." University Honors Thesis, paper 818, 2019. https://doi.org/10.15760/honors.837.

Chapter 7: How to Ask for What You Want

1 "Desire is to own the wanting. It is a claim: I *want*": Perel, Esther in interview with Monica Padman and Jess Rowland. "Monica & Jess Love Goblins with Esther Perel" (Part 7). *Monica & Jess Love Boys*, March 25, 2020. Simplecast, Armchair Expert Podcast. https://armchairexpertpod.com/pods/mjlb-esther-perel.

2 "Rejection is protection": Chase, Elle. *Curvy Girl Sex: 101 Body-Positive Positions to Empower Your Sex Life*. Beverly, MA: Fair Winds, 2017.

3 non-monogamy has evolved: Ryan, Christopher. *Sex at Dawn: How We Mate, Why We Stray, and What It Means for Modern Relationships*. New York; Harper Perennial, 2012; Perel, Esther. *Mating in Captivity: Reconciling the Erotic and the Domestic*. New York: HarperCollins, 2009.

4 in relationship to others: Cacioppo, John T., and William Patrick. *Loneliness: Human Nature and the Need for Social Connection*. New York: W. W. Norton & Company, 2008.

5 pack mentality: Bloom, Howard K. *Global Brain: The Evolution of Mass Mind from the Big Bang to the 21st Century*. New York: John Wiley, 2001.

6 comfort in predictable patterns: Ersche, Karen D., Tsen-Vei Lim, Laetitia H. E. Ward, Trevor W. Robbins, and Jan Stochl. "Creature of Habit: A Self-Report Measure of Habitual Routines and Automatic Tendencies in Everyday Life." *Personality and Individual Differences* 116 (2017): 73–85. https://doi.org/10.1016/j.paid.2017.04.024.

7 fight, flight, freeze, or fawn: Walker, Pete. *Complex PTSD: From Surviving to Thriving: A Guide and Map for Recovering from Childhood Trauma*. Lafayette, CA: Azure Coyote, 2013.

8 negativity bias: Rozin, Paul, and Edward B. Royzman. "Negativity Bias, Negativity Dominance, and Contagion." *Personality and Social*

Psychology Review 5, no. 4 (2001): 296–320. https://doi.org/10.1207 /s15327957pspr0504_2.

9 linked to depression and anxiety: Primack, Brian A., Meghan A. Bisbey, Ariel Shensa, Nicholas D. Bowman, Sabrina A. Karim, Jennifer M. Knight, and Jaime E. Sidani. "The Association between Valence of Social Media Experiences and Depressive Symptoms." *Depression and Anxiety* 35, no. 8 (2018): 784–94. https://doi.org/10.1002/da.22779.

10 face the door: Halliday, Ayun. "The Power of Conformity: 1962 Episode of *Candid Camera* Reveals the Strange Psychology of Riding Elevators." Open Culture, November 7, 2016. https://www .openculture.com/2016/11/the-power-of-conformity-1962-episode -of-candid-camera-reveals-the-psychology-of-riding-elevators.html.

11 fundamentally safe and healthy: "Healthy vs. Unhealthy Relationships." The University of Alabama Counseling Center. Retrieved April 15, 2020. https://counseling.sa.ua.edu/resources/healthy-vs-unhealthy -relationships.

12 "Rejection is protection": Chase, Elle. *Curvy Girl Sex: 101 Body-Positive Positions to Empower Your Sex Life*. Beverly, MA: Fair Winds, 2017.

13 dopamine is flowing: Raz, Guy in interview with Helen Fisher. "What Happen to Our Brain When We're in Love?" April 25, 2014. Ted Radio Hour, NPR.

Chapter 8: Setting Your Sexual Boundaries

1 "risk disappointing others": Brown, Brené. *Daring Greatly: How the Courage to Be Vulnerable Transforms the Way We Live, Love, Parent, and Lead*. New York: Avery, 2012.

2 "'Fuck Yes' sex": Manson, Mark. "Fuck Yes or No." Mark Manson, July 8, 2013. https://markmanson.net/fuck-yes.

3 a recurrence of a traumatic event: Van der Kolk, Bessel. *The Body Keeps the Score: Brain, Mind and Body in the Healing of Trauma*. New York: Penguin Books, 2015.

4 book about sex: See my favorite recommendations in the resource guide.

5 handy lists: "Needs Inventory." Center for Nonviolent Communication, 2005. https://www.cnvc.org/training/resource/needs-inventory.

6 risk disappointing others: Brown, Brené. *Daring Greatly: How the Courage to Be Vulnerable Transforms the Way We Live, Love, Parent, and Lead*. New York: Avery, 2012.

7 good, statistical reasons: "National Statistics Domestic Violence Fact Sheet." National Coalition Against Domestic Violence, 2020. https://ncadv.org/STATISTICS.

Chapter 9: How to Hear No Like a Pro

1 *differentiation*: Titelman, Peter. *Differentiation of Self: Bowen Family Systems Theory Perspectives*. New York: Routledge, 2015.

2 Murray Bowen in the 1950s: Kerr, Michael E. "Bowen Theory and Therapy." In: *The Handbook of Marriage and Marital Therapy*, ed. G. Pirooz Sholevar (143–72). Berlin: Springer, 1981. https://doi.org/10.1007/978-94-017-3340-3_6.

3 Developmental Model of Couples Therapy: The Developmental Model of Couples Therapy and differentiation are easily digestible in Winifred M. Reilly's book *It Takes One to Tango* and slightly less digestible but extremely applicable to one's sex life in David Schnarch's famous book *Passionate Marriage*.

4 Ellyn Bader and Peter Pearson: Bader, Ellyn, and Peter T. Pearson. *In Quest of the Mythical Mate: A Developmental Approach to Diagnosis and Treatment in Couples Therapy*. London: Routledge, 2014.

5 Developmental Model of Couples Therapy: Bader, Ellyn, and Peter T. Pearson. *In Quest of the Mythical Mate: A Developmental Approach to Diagnosis and Treatment in Couples Therapy*. London: Routledge, 2014.

6 four distinct relationship stages: Bader, Ellyn, and Peter T. Pearson. *In Quest of the Mythical Mate: A Developmental Approach to Diagnosis and Treatment in Couples Therapy*. London: Routledge, 2014.

7 *new relationship energy*: Dagger, Jesse. "We've All Been There: Common NRE Mistakes." Polyamory for Us, September 15, 2020. https://www.polyfor.us/articles/common-nre-mistakes.

8 oxytocin: Algoe, Sara B., Laura E. Kurtz, and Karen Grewen. "Oxytocin and Social Bonds: The Role of Oxytocin in Perceptions of Romantic Partners' Bonding Behavior." *Psychological Science* 28, no. 12 (2017): 1763–72. https://doi.org/10.1177/0956797617716922.

9 *vitality*: Bader, Ellyn, and Peter T. Pearson. *In Quest of the Mythical Mate: A Developmental Approach to Diagnosis and Treatment in Couples Therapy*. London: Routledge, 2014.

10 shooting for: In the four-phase model of Bader and Pearson's Developmental Model of Couples Therapy, Figure 3 shows stages 3 and 4—Exploration and Rapprochement.

11 simply being asexual: Conley-Fonda, Brenna, and Taylor Leisher. "Asexuality: Sexual Health Does Not Require Sex." *Sexual Addiction & Compulsivity* 25, no. 1 (2018): 6–11. https://doi.org/10.1080/107201 62.2018.1475699.

12 "Consent and Cookies": Tallon-Hicks, Yana. "Consent & Cookies: A Confidence-Building Workshop for Teens." Yana Tallon-Hicks, October 11, 2018. https://yanatallonhicks.com/workshops/for-youth /consent-for-teens.

13 "Curious, Not Furious": Bader, and Peter Pearson in interview with Neil Sattin. "Why We Lie and How to Get Back to the Truth with Ellyn Bader and Peter Pearson" (episode). Relationship Alive!, February 23, 2016. Podcast. https://www.neilsattin.com /blog/2016/02/24-why-we-lie-and-how-to-get-back-to-the-truth with-ellyn-bader-and-peter-pearson.

Chapter 10: How to Repair a Boundary Mistake

1 "in a state of shame": Roth, Lea and Stas Schmiedt. "How Shame Can Block Accountability." Barnard Center for Research on Women, October 10, 2019. YouTube video. https://www.youtube.com /watch?v=58nAd6gDZKA.

2 "'I believe you can transform'": brown, adrienne maree. "What Is Transformative Justice?"Barnard Center for Research on Women, 2021. Produced by Mariame Kaba, Dean Spade, and Hope Dector. Vimeo. https://vimeo.com/395756782.

3 will experience sexual assault: "Victims of Sexual Violence: Statistics." RAINN, 2020. https://www.rainn.org/statistics/victims -sexual-violence.

4 one in 33 (presumed cisgender) men: "Victims of Sexual Violence: Statistics." RAINN, 2020. https://www.rainn.org/statistics/victims -sexual-violence.

5 in their lifetime: James, S. E., J. L. Herman, S. Rankin, M. Keisling, L. Mottet, and M. Anafi. *"Executive Summary of the Report of the 2015 U.S. Transgender Survey."* Washington, DC: National Center for Transgender Equality, 2016.

6 highly disproportionately affected: James, S. E., J. L. Herman, S. Rankin, M. Keisling, L. Mottet, and M. Anafi. *"Executive Summary of the Report of the 2015 U.S. Transgender Survey."* Washington, DC: National Center for Transgender Equality, 2016.

7 bodies respond physiologically to it: Michl, Petra, Thomas Meindl, Franziska Meister, Christine Born, Rolf R. Engel, Maximilian Reiser, and Kristina Hennig-Fast. "Neurobiological Underpinnings of Shame and Guilt: A Pilot FMRI Study." *Social Cognitive and Affective Neuroscience* 9, no. 2 (2012): 150–57. https://doi.org/10.1093/scan/nss114.

8 "Guilt is 'I did something bad.'": Brown, Brené. "Listening to Shame." TED, March 2012. https://www.ted.com/talks/brene_brown _listening_to_shame.

9 wider transformative justice: "Transformative Justice is a political framework and approach for responding to violence, harm and abuse. At its most basic, it seeks to respond to violence without creating more violence. . . . Transformative justice responses and interventions 1) do not rely on the state . . . ; 2) do not reinforce or perpetuate violence such as oppressive norms or vigilantism; and most importantly, 3) actively cultivate the things we know prevent violence such as healing, accountability, resilience, and safety for all involved." Mingus, Mia. "Transformative Justice: A Brief Description." TransformHarm.org, 2020. https://transformharm.org/transformative -justice-a-brief-description. For more reading on transformative justice, see the resource guide.

10 Call-in: Trần, Ngọc Loan. "Calling IN: A Less Disposable Way of Holding Each Other Accountable." *BGD* (blog), December 18, 2013. https://www.bgdblog.org/2013/12/calling-less-disposable -way-holding-accountable.

11 get to safety: "Create a Safety Plan: Interactive Guide to Safety Planning." National Domestic Violence Hotline, Accessed September 27, 2020. https://www.thehotline.org/plan-for-safety/create-a-safety-plan.

12 Karina Schumann published her research findings: Schumann, Karina. "An Affirmed Self and a Better Apology: The Effect of

Self-Affirmation on Transgressors' Responses to Victims." *Journal of Experimental Social Psychology* 54 (2014): 89–96. https://doi.org/10.1016/j.jesp.2014.04.013.

13 contextually set up: Lefkowitz, Eva S., and Tara M. Stoppa. "Positive Sexual Communication and Socialization in the Parent-Adolescent Context." *New Directions for Child and Adolescent Development* 2006, no. 112 (2006): 39–55. https://doi.org/10.1002/cd.161.

14 an accountability process: T. K. "Accountability Process Primer." F12 Network, June 5, 2017. https://f12network.wordpress.com/accountability-process-primer.

15 an accountability buddy-system: Crimethinc. "Thinking Through Perpetrator Accountability." TransformHarm.org, March 1, 2021. https://transformharm.org/thinking-through-perpetrator-accountability.

16 traditional BDSM color system: Dunkley, Cara R., and Lori A. Brotto. "The Role of Consent in the Context of BDSM." *Sexual Abuse* 32, no. 6 (2019): 657–78. https://doi.org/10.1177/1079063219842847.

Chapter 11: How to Navigate Desire Discrepancies (When Your Yes Is Their No)

1 gridlock is to move: Reilly, Winifred M. *It Takes One to Tango*. New York: Simon & Schuster, 2017.

2 narrative therapy: Carr, Alan. "Michael White's Narrative Therapy." *Contemporary Family Therapy* 20 (1998): 485–503.

3 externalizing interview: Ackerman, Courtney E. "19 Narrative Therapy Techniques, Interventions + Worksheets." PositivePsychology.com, April 15, 2021. https://positivepsychology.com/narrative-therapy.

ABOUT THE AUTHOR

Yana Tallon-Hicks, LMFT, is a sex therapist specializing in LGBTQQ+, kinky, and non-monogamous relationships. She is also a consent, sex, and sexuality columnist and educator. Whether written or with clients, her work centers around the belief that pleasure-positive and consent-based sex education can positively impact our lives and the world. She lives in western Massachusetts. For more about Yana and her practice, visit her website at yanatallonhicks.com or follow her on Instagram @the_vspot.

ABOUT THE ILLUSTRATOR

Rebeca Soto is a queer Chicana erotic illustrator from Chicago. Her mixed-media artwork aims to celebrate sexual liberation through an illustrated feminist lens. Intimate moments and sensual spectrums take shape through her digital dreamscapes, painted portraits, and full-color stories. Enjoy the details of her figures and fantasy spaces at rebecasoto.com.